To Nancy,
Thanks for your support

Dominick P. Varsalone, RN

# My Journey as an AIDS Nurse

D1569180

# My Journey as an AIDS Nurse

DOMINICK P VARSALONE AND SALLY DEERING

ISBN: 1539752011
ISBN 13: 9781539752011
Library of Congress Control Number: 2016918041
CreateSpace Independent Publishing Platform
North Charleston, South Carolina

"When AIDS is stopped we will dance for joy.
Until then we will dance for life."

- D. J.

# Table of Contents

# One

## 1995
## Da' Bomb

It's my first evening as an AIDS Nurse at Broadway House in Newark and I'm at the nurses' station when the telephone rings. I pick it up and a male voice on the line says. "There is a bomb in an attaché case under the piano in the rotunda. I put it there to kill all the AIDS -infected faggots and the bitches that care for them."

He hangs up and I go pale. I call the nursing supervisor and she meets me in the rotunda scared to death. We edge over to the piano and there's the attaché case right where he said it would be.

The nursing supervisor whispers to me to go to each unit and tell all the nurses and nursing assistants to gather the patients who can walk and get them to the first floor of the West Wing. This area is far away from the attaché case and next to an exit door. Then she calls the Newark Police Department and tells them we are in "Code: Yellow". We are instructed to take all the residents outside to the nursing home on the other side of the building. Some are confined to their beds, so we take them bed and all. Meanwhile, there's a torrential downpour outside.

1

Police cars show up and park facing the building, but the cops don't attempt to get out, they just sit in their cars. Not one policeman comes inside to talk or help us. They know this is a hospice that houses AIDS patients and they don't go inside for fear they'll catch something. They won't even hold the doors open for us as we wheel the patients to safety.

The bomb squad arrives and steps out of their cars wearing gloves. They proceed to put on black vests and helmets for protection. We wait at the nursing home next door. The bomb squad opens the case and finds two D-batteries taped to wires. It's not a bomb. They give the "all clear" and we quickly get all the patients back to their rooms. The police take off without so much as a good-bye.

What have I gotten myself into?

# 1986
# First Baseman Bob

It was early on in the 1986 New York City softball season, and I was one of the team members fielding calls from new players. One of the new guys was Bob Buhr who had just moved to Brooklyn from Chicago. He was a first baseman and we needed a first baseman.

Okay, I have to tell you right up front that my initial attraction to Bob was very strong. He was tall – about six feet – slim, with thick brown hair, the most beautiful blue eyes and a great smile.

I was a team coach, but there was nothing I had to coach Bob about, he immediately became one of our best players.

About two or three games into the season, I don't think we had won a game yet, I noticed a woman I had never seen before talking to everyone on the team like she knew them. I found out she was Bob's friend Millie from Chicago, and had taken a few days off to visit him in New York. While the game was going on she was right there with the rest of the team, interviewing guys she thought would be a good dating prospect for Bob. Apparently Bob had been in New York almost six months and was so focused on his new job that he never bothered to socialize. Bob knew no one other than colleagues from work he occasionally met for dinner.

Millie was about to change that. I mean this woman had a pad and pencil and was taking notes. She "interviewed" most of the team except me, and when I asked why, she said, "Bob wanted you on the list but you are with someone". I told her I was single (I had just broken up with someone) and she immediately added my name.

After the game, we all went back to our host bar, the Barbary Coast on 7th Avenue and 14th Street. I saw Millie and Bob at the bar and went over to talk. I told them a little bit about my situation and how I was unsure if I wanted to date right now, but I was also very happy to be on Millie's list of potentials.

I asked how long Millie was going to be in town, and she told me she would be leaving the next day. I asked how she was getting to the airport and Bob said that since he didn't have a car, they would take public transportation. In my usual style, I stepped right up and asked if they wanted me to pick them up and take them to the airport in my van. Simultaneously, Bob said "no" and Millie responded "yes".

Millie won.

After we dropped Millie off for her flight home, I asked Bob if he had any plans for the rest of the day and he said, "no not really, I was just planning to go home and relax." Of course

I wanted to go with him and show him how I like to relax on Sunday afternoons with a hot guy, but it was Mother's Day and every year my mom and I celebrated Mother's Day and my birthday together. I could not let Mom down, so I did the next best thing. I invited Bob to my parents' house in Jersey City where he would meet my entire family.

When we arrived. I introduced Bob and it seemed as though everyone felt immediately comfortable and also relieved because no one in my family liked my ex-boyfriend. Bob also seemed to be right at home with my family. Our first photo together is a picture of us playing with my nieces Tara and Allison and my nephew, Nick.

Before we left, I had to wash some clothes in my mom's basement, so before we went upstairs to say goodnight to everyone, we spent a few minutes by the washing machine testing out the first gay requirement of a new relationship: kissing. If he's a good kisser, you can move forward; if not, you may be looking at another two-week relationship.

## Bowling Buddies

After Bob and I were dating regularly, we joined the NYC Gay Men's Bowling League, and the couple we most connected with was Cal and Frankie. Cal was tall, with sandy brown hair; very handsome. His eyes were blue, beautiful and sincere, like Bob's.

It was Christmas 1986 and Cal and Frankie invited Bob and I to their apartment on 24th Street in Union Square for a party where we met their close friends. You know how you go to a party and there are some people there you just know you will be friends with forever? Clearly, all their friends were top-notch with no pretense.

4

Cal worked for Leona Helmsley at her hotel "The Helmsley Palace" on 5th Avenue and he had the greatest work stories like when he and five co-workers were setting up the ballroom for a grand party at Helmsley Palace. Leona had three men and three women doing all the preparations. When Leona entered the room in her high-falutin' fashion, she started screaming, "no, no, no! This is all wrong! This is not what I asked for."

Pointing to the three women, she said, "you, you and you – OUT." Gesturing to Cal and his two co-workers – both gay – who stood there not knowing what to do, Leona snapped her fingers and said, "you three fix this!" Then she stormed out of the room.

Immediately after finishing the story, Frankie, who had been playing Christmas carols on their Baby Grand Piano started singing, "We three Queens for Leona work ..." Everybody cracked up.

Cal said Leona was real tough to work for, but she did love the gay boys and I think the gay boys loved her because she was fierce, just like those old movie stars Bette Davis, Joan Crawford and Tallulah Bankhead.

Frankie was shorter than Cal and well-built. He was a dancer, had his own dance company. Frankie was so Italian he made me look like a WASP.

Cal was one of the founders of the Gotham Open Gay Bowling Tournament. Cal bowled competitively and had close to a 200-average; his team was always one of the best in the league.

## Could it Be GRID?

When Bob and I moved into our new apartment in Jersey City, Cal and Frankie came for dinner. I had the worst cold and sore throat and Cal was telling me he had just gotten over a cold. I remember we talked about the "gay plague" that was going around. It was frightening in those days because every time you got the slightest cold you thought you were going to get really sick and die.

It was soon to be 1987, and in the last six years many people we knew had died very quickly from this mysterious virus, taken from us way too soon. We talked about how we were in relationships and it would not affect us because it was usually the single guys who had multiple sex partners – they were the ones more likely to get the gay plague.

During this time, TV stations and other media outlets put out news stories about Gay Related Immune Deficiency (GRID) almost daily. In the gay community, any place gay men congregated, activists were there delivering the most up-to-date information on GRID. These activists saved the lives of many who took their advice and educated themselves. Unfortunately, the government under President Ronald Reagan ignored the reports, turned its head away and kept silent. The blood of many of my dear friends is on Reagan's hands and the hands of New York City Mayor Ed Koch who allegedly was a gay man locked in the closet. Koch ignored the news reports about gay men dying at a rapid rate in New York City, the city Koch supposedly loved so much. The city that, as mayor, Koch swore to protect.

In 1987 – a year later – the New York gay community organized and formed Act-Up New York. That's the year I joined.

From September of 1987 through the holidays and into 1988, Cal had been hospitalized three times. Bob and I didn't know if Cal had GRID or a flu he couldn't shake. I think deep down we knew the truth, but we couldn't admit it was happening to someone we cared so much about. We were in denial.

Cal was in Beth Israel Hospital in New York in September and then again in November, but he was doing a little better, so he and Frankie held their holiday party on Christmas Eve. Bob and I arrived and Frankie greeted us at the door dressed in his tuxedo. Cal was holding court in a lounge chair to the side. He also was wearing a tux minus the jacket. We saw he was also wearing a cast. I asked why and he laughed. Frankie explained that Cal was feeling pretty good in comparison to the last few months when they were decorating for the party. Cal was making fun of Frankie dancing when he slipped and fell and broke his arm trying to catch the fall. It was the highlight of the party. We all sat around trying to decorate Cal and his cast. It was the best party I had ever been to. They both looked so handsome. Cal was feeling great, he said, and looked it, too.

# 1989
## One Last Dance

On Valentines Day, Cal and Frankie decided they would have a couples-only party. Cal was getting frail after his third bout of PCP. (Pneumocystis Carinii Pneumonia is a serious infection of the lungs that often affects people with HIV/AIDS). Cal and Frankie wanted to throw this party for their special friends. By the end of the night it was pretty clear that Cal was not going to make it to Christmas.

One Friday evening in September, I met Bob in the New York City and we went to see Cal for the last time. Cal was on a respirator and it was so hard to see him like that. Bob and I could not hold back our tears. Frankie was so strong, that night; he somehow got us through it all.

Taking one last look at Cal before we left, I prayed to God to please pull him through, but I knew in my heart that our dear friend had no more miracles left.

We got the call Saturday evening that Cal had died at 2:30 that afternoon. I wrote in my diary that night. "My dear friend Cal, we love you, we will miss you and we will take good care of Frankie for you."

Cal and Frankie were our favorite couple to be with, and now we were forming a different kind of friendship with Frankie; and it was deep and very special.

Bob helped Frankie with all the paperwork on finances and wills and we spent a lot of time together for the rest of that year. In our many conversations with Frankie, we came to the conclusion that what we would miss most about Cal would be the annual holiday party he threw with Frankie. Frankie told us he could not bring himself to do it anymore, so Bob and I decided to honor our friends by becoming the hosts of the holiday party.

When Christmas rolled around, we kept our promise and about 70 people showed up. Frankie was not able to make the party though because he was invited to be with Cal's family that year in Pennsylvania. Everyone had a great time, there was plenty food, drink, and Bob's home-baked goodies. There was, however, still a bit of heaviness in the air, as the conversations turned to shared memories of our friends who had passed away from AIDS. The following year there were many more friends who died, and Frankie told us he too was infected. We spent as much time with Frankie that year when he was feeling well and also when he was not.

# 1991
# I Should Be What?

I'm at St. Vincent Hospital in Greenwich Village to see my friend Frankie. His family and friends set up a visitation schedule so he would never be alone. Frankie became really sick in mid-February; he was in end-stage AIDS.

His room was in a unit of 12 negative-pressure rooms each occupied by an end-stage AIDS patient. In order to see him, I had to put on yellow protective gear.

When I entered the room, and took his hand, Frankie was frantically trying to tell me something. "I have guelph!" he stated rather emphatically.

"Guelph" I thought, I had no idea what that is. What was he trying to tell me? I kept asking him over and over again, what is Guelph? Finally, because he was soiled, I said "do you mean diarrhea?" and he threw his arms up and shook his head "yes."

I didn't know what to do, at first. There was only one nurse on the floor and she was all the way down the hall. I went to tell her Frankie had soiled himself, and she told me that he wasn't a priority at the moment, that she had to hang patients' IVs, dole out pain medication, and give injections. All that was way more important than one patient's diarrhea. Other people are dying in the unit, she said, and she was the only nurse on duty.

I said to her, "Okay, show me where the supplies are and I'll do it."

She smiled and pointed to the linen closet down the hall. I went back to Frankie's room and cleaned him up. I have no idea what even made me think that I could complete a task like that, but I thank God for giving me the strength and ability, and I thank the nurse – I wish I remembered her name – for allowing me to assist.

Later, she came into Frankie's room to check on him. He was resting. She turned to me and asked: "Are you a nurse?"

"Me? A nurse? Oh no," I told her.

"What do you do for a living?" she asked.

"I'm an unemployed freight train repairman," I told her.

Looking puzzled, she said, "You should be a nurse. We could use you here,"

She hugged me, and left the room to continue her work.

I went back to Frankie's bedside and I was stroking his hair not knowing if he was too sick to hear what she just said. "Imagine that," I whispered to him, "she thinks I should be a nurse. What do you think? Frankie?"

For a minute he was still and had no response. A few minutes of silence passed then I noticed Frankie nodding his head up and down, "yes!"

## The Promise

The following Saturday, Valentine's Day, I went to the florist on Monmouth Street in Jersey City, owned by a young lady named Dawn G. I have always loved flowers and plants, who doesn't, but all through my life flowers have had a significant impact on what direction I was headed. I walked into this little flower shop and Dawn said to me, "Are you looking for Valentine flowers for your wife?"

"No," I said with a chuckle, "my husband."

Dawn laughed. She had the cutest laugh.

She had a sign posted on the wall, "Last Valentine's Day for Dawn's Flower Shop."

"It's your last day?" I asked.

"Yes," she said. "Next year will be my senior year at Christ Hospital School of Nursing and I can't do both anymore."

"I've been thinking of going to nursing school, too," I said. "My friend is in the hospital with AIDS and his nurse encouraged me to go."

I could see her eyes welling up with tears, so I gave her a hug.

"Do it!' she said. "Go to nursing school."

I left with flowers, but I don't remember paying for them. Dawn was a messenger sent by God; and the message was clear.

# Tiny Dancer

Frankie was in ICU and visitation was family only, and since I wasn't family, I couldn't visit. I was working a temporary job as a deliveryman for Minuteman Press and the following week I had to make a delivery to Christ Hospital School of Nursing in Jersey City. I ran into the Public Affairs Director Barbara Davey and said, "May I have a nursing school application for my sister?" I did not want her to know it was really for me.

I was telling Barbara how I was filling in for a driver who had suffered a heart attack and that I was looking for a new direction since losing my job. Barbara said, "Why don't you pick up a nursing school application for yourself, too?" Off I went to my next delivery stop with two nursing school applications in hand.

My sister and I filled out our applications together. I turned them in the very next day and was told that in order to get in for the fall term in September, we had to take the entrance test in March. Just before the test date, my sister found out she was pregnant again and said: "I don't want to be in nursing school and pregnant at the same time."

I went back to Dawn's Flower Shop and she gave me all the information I needed, plus a boost of confidence, and her cute laugh.

"Do it;" she said. "You will be a great nurse."

Bob and I were getting ready to sit down to dinner that night when the phone rang. It was Frankie's brother telling us Frankie passed away peacefully that day, surrounded by family. His brother said his funeral would be private, but before the end of March, they would empty the apartment. Frankie wanted Bob and I to have the Baby Grand piano.

Two weeks later, we were at Frankie's apartment with his family to help them move everything out. It was surreal as we watched the piano movers move Frankie's Baby Grand to our house in Jersey City.

This devastating loss almost stopped me dead in my tracks.

A week later, I took the entrance exam at Christ Hospital School of Nursing. The test was so difficult; I thought I would never pass. I went to the chapel at St. Francis Hospital to say a prayer. "God," I said, "if you help me pass this test, I promise I will be the best nurse I can be."

# TWO

## 1996
## Gonna Take a Miracle

It's a very cold February morning and I arrive at Broadway House early, as usual. I've been working here six months now; the beds are filled in every unit and there's a waiting list to get in. There's even talk of renovating the West Wing storage areas and turning the space into patient rooms.

After the morning report from the midnight shift charge nurse, and hearing that there was another death the night before, I take a seat in the office and wait for the next admission. It's a pretty grave situation. Edgar, an 18 year-old with AIDS, jumped out his apartment window to kill himself, but failed. He's dealing with AIDS and complications from his injuries.

Meanwhile, since I've been at Broadway House, they promoted me to assistant charge nurse. So I call in my staff for a short meeting and let them know about Edgar. The hospital ambulance arrives and brings him to his room. His older sister Juanita follows with two small children. I let them all settle in and say a little prayer before I enter with my clipboard and pen. I walk in and the two little girls are playing with dolls and Juanita sits in a chair crying next to Edgar's bed. I introduce myself.

"Good morning, my name is Dominick and I am Edgar's nurse today." I knew from his hospital chart that Edgar is aphasic (a communication disorder resulting from damage to the part of the brain that contains language) so I know he can't respond verbally.

Theresa and Beverly are the CNA's, (Certified Nursing Assistants) working with me today, and Ms. Shirley is the LPN. I ask them to come in to tend to Edgar while I talk with his sister. They do a phenomenal job cleaning him and making him feel as comfortable as possible. Juanita is still crying, so I go over to comfort her. I ask if it would be okay to bring the two little girls to the activity room where a therapist can look after them while we talk; she nods "yes."

I sit face-to-face with Juanita and take her hands in mine. I ask her to explain in her words what she's feeling, and details about what happened to her brother. She says, "Edgar is my brother and I love him, but he has AIDS because he is gay and God is punishing him for it."

I look her right in the eyes and say, "what you believe is your choice. Who your brother is, well, that's who God made him to be. We can't choose to be gay. We are born this way. There is no choice."

I hold her hands firmly, and I think she begins to realize she is talking and holding hands with a gay man. I want her to get that message and I think she does.

"Do you want your brother to recover from this or do you see this as the end for him?" I ask her.

"No," she says, "I want him to get better, but I don't think he wants to live anymore."

I ask her to tell him she loves him and that it will be okay if he fights to get better. The message I'm trying to convey to her is that she should focus on being his sister, not his judge or preacher.

I know she got my message, and I leave her alone with her brother for a short time and return to began my assessment. Since Edgar is aphasic, I use the hand-squeezing method of communication: one squeeze for "yes" and two squeezes for "no". Looking directly into his eyes is imperative.

I ask Edgar a series of health-related questions and he does a great job of answering them. I tell him about my conversation with his sister and about the new Protease Inhibitors coming out. I let him know that if he wants a chance at getting better we will do our best to help him. I also want him to know that if he does not want to fight, we will do our best to make him comfortable and as free from pain as possible. My last question is the most important and will determine his plan of care.

"Do you want to let us help you try to fight this battle?" I ask.

Edgar squeezes my hand I look at him, "Are you sure?" He squeezes again.

One time for "yes".

I return to my office, and put my head in my arms to think – and yes – to cry, a little. I sit there knowing I could not promise Edgar the Protease Inhibitors would make him better, but I know that fighting the battle with *a will to live* will take him halfway there.

I write up an extensive care plan for Edgar including routine care that is given to every patient. However, Edgar needs more than most patients. His plan includes wound care three times a day, and range-of-motion exercises every two hours to help him become mobile again. His body is contracted. He also has a feeding tube.

I know the CNAs will have to work extra hard to care for Edgar and they are as ready for the challenge as I am. They even give him the nickname "Baby Boy" because he's so young, the youngest patient we've treated so far. I add a full body massage with lotion three times a day to his treatment plan.

When I present this care plan at the care plan meeting, everyone says I'm crazy. Our unit social worker, Gloria thinks its a great plan and tells me she will do everything she can to make it happen. Every hospital discipline has made a commitment to make this work and we are ready to start moving – of course, with the doctor's approval.

Very often our physicians are unable to do their assessment the same day the patient arrives, but our rule is that within 24 hours a physician assessment must be completed. The next day, Dr. Moaven arrives to do Edgar's assessment.

I have a tremendous amount of respect for Dr. M and I am excited to tell him my plan of care for Edgar. I do paperwork while the doctor is in with Edgar. When he finishes his report he knocks on my door to give me his paperwork. He plops it on my desk and says, "I give this one two-weeks."

Stunned by his remark I say, "Excuse me, what do you mean by that?" He cautiously says to me, "He's in really bad shape, Dominick." Dr. M knows me, and changing his tune he says, "What do you have in mind?"

I stand up so I can be eye-to-eye with him and I give him my assessment and how Edgar himself told me through non-verbal communication that he wants to fight and get better. I show him my care plan and ask him to put Edgar on the newly approved three-drug regimen of Protease Inhibitors and allow us to initiate this challenge.

Dr. M smiles at me and says, "Whatever you want Dominick, you're the best."

"No doctor, we're the best. It is going to take a very dedicated team to make this happen, and I thank you for your confidence in me."

He shakes my hand and walks out of my office. A new day dawns for Edgar.

In the weeks that follow, Edgar not only survives, he thrives. Every day he is moving more, slowly, but with improvement. When he first arrived his T-cell count was in the single digits and his viral load was over a million. He could not walk or talk except with non-verbal communication and he was what we considered a "total care patient". Edgar is working very hard day and night and becoming stronger every day.

Three weeks after the new medication was administered, we perform more blood work to see if it was effective. Three weeks after that the results are in and they are remarkable. In addition to that good news, the CNAs have Edgar standing in the doorway not quite walking on his own but still, this is nothing short of a miracle.

Edgar's family is amazed with his progress and his sister Juanita visits often. She always thanks us for giving her brother back to the world of those who are "living with AIDS."

My next promise to Edgar is that if he's able to walk on his own without an assistive device before the end of June, I will take him to the Gay Pride Parade in New York City. Edgar tells me he has never seen the Gay Pride Parade, so it gives him something to work for. Soon the feeding tube is removed and he has gained weight. Every staff member wants to feed him goodies and he loves the attention.

Edgar talks, too, although not in his usual full voice. Soon he is able to walk, although he has a permanent limp.

Dr. M calls him, "Our Broadway Miracle."

He is my first miracle at Broadway House.

# 1991
# Grandpa Nightingale

I think I can speak for every nurse when I say nursing school is hell; I've yet to meet a nurse who said she or he breezed through nursing school without at least one panic attack. I had mine the minute I walked through the entrance door to Christ Hospital School of Nursing in Jersey City, a very old, traditional nursing school that's been around since 1890.

It was September 1991. When I walked through the foyer of Christ Hospital School of Nursing, the very walls of the building seemed to be "screaming", "What the hell are you doing here?" That's exactly how I felt.

I entered the main lobby that was painted a dark green and lined with photographs of graduates from years past, rows of nurses in white uniforms holding red roses. Some of the pictures were so old they were in black and white with the nurses dressed in crisp white dresses and huge nursing caps trimmed with two rows of black ribbon. Aside from the uniforms and the nurses' stoic, unsmiling faces, the only difference between the then and now pictures was that there were no men until the class of 1990. I now understand why no one in any of the pictures was smiling. They were exhausted.

Other first-year students gathered in the lobby and the little side waiting room, again with the green walls and furniture that looked like it came from grandma's attic – big, overstuffed chairs, a loveseat couch, end tables and frilly white curtains on the windows. The only thing missing were doilies on the arm rests. My first thought was that if I failed at nursing they might want to hire me as the new interior decorator. This place needed a little bit of the gay touch.

There were a lot of us lingering in the hall and spilling into that tiny waiting room, making small talk, until Brenda Pellicano, the secretary, and Cathe Killman, the House Mother came to greet us.

"Good morning Class of 1994 and welcome to Christ Hospital School of Nursing," she said to the group. "If you will all assemble in the first floor classroom, we can get this day started."

When I first met Ms. Killman, visions of Kathy Bates went through my mind. With a name like Killman I was happy I was not going to board at the school dormitory. It turns out that Ms. Killman was the sweetest woman anyone could know. I showed her respect right from the beginning and she loved me right to the end. My first lesson in why we should not pass judgment!

We walked down the hall and entered the classroom; a dilapidated room painted a dull gray and brightly lit with fluorescent lights that made me squint. We took our seats in old school desks with the tops that folded to the side. I looked around and noticed almost everyone else was younger than me except one woman who I thought was one of the instructors. I felt like a 35 year-old on his first day of Kindergarten.

There were 75 of us crammed in that room: 18 men – mostly young Filipinos – and me, looking like the daddy of them all. (In 1991, less than 5 percent of all nurses were men. Most male nurses were either military, or worked in the Emergency Room (ER) and Operating Room (OR). Suddenly a stream of people walked in single file and the first thing that came to mind was that they should be playing "Hail to the Chief," on the overhead speakers. They introduced themselves.

"Hello Class of 1994. My name is Carol Fasano and I'm the Director of Nursing," she said.

A few others spoke and described their roles in our education process; I was focused on the only man in that line, wondering how he survives in a female-dominated work environment. Then it was his turn.

"Hello Class of 1994, I'm George Hebert, RN, and Assistant Director of Nursing."

I felt somewhat relieved and looked forward to sitting down with Mr. Hebert and learning more about how a man makes it in nursing. Since I was coming from an all-male profession into a female-dominated profession, it was important to get his input on how a man copes.

In the past, when I worked with all-men, our conversations during breaks were what we would be getting our wives and girl-friends for Christmas. What will it be like working with so many women? I never gave a thought as to whether Mr. Hebert was straight or gay at that time, but then other questions started pop-ping up in my head. Do I tell my classmates about my personal life? Should I let them in? Knowing I'm gay, will they accept me? And if I don't say anything, will they just assume I'm gay because I'm a man in nursing?

I realized I was a double-minority: a man in a female-dominated profession and the only one in my class who identi-fied as an openly gay man. At least I thought I was the only one.

All the instructors stepped up to the front of the class, and introduced themselves. I wondered which one would be my clini-cal instructor. Most seemed rigid, about as flexible as the iron bars I worked with on the railroad. Others seemed like they were compassionate, but they were stifling their compassion because they didn't want to portray any vulnerability to the students. It was like being at boot camp. Many of them were my age or even younger, which made me a little uncomfortable.

Our class advisor, Joanne Growney addressed the class.

"Now students, you should know that about 50 percent of the students in this room will not make it through the first year of nursing school."

I immediately thought I would be one of them. Should I just leave now?

Mrs. Growney said, "Our job is to make good compassionate nurses out of all of you."

Now that everyone was introduced, the Director of Nursing Carol Fasano addressed all of us.

"The curriculum for first year nursing students is broken into six semesters. In the first semester, we begin with the Fundamentals of Nursing or Nursing 101. You will be receiving your textbooks by the end of the day and you are required to read the first 22 chapters for class tomorrow. There is nothing like getting started right away eh?"

I don't think I have ever read 22 chapters of anything in my whole life.

"We will meet in the Skills Lab located in the basement first thing in the morning. Thank you and again, welcome to Christ Hospital."

The administrators took us on a tour of the school, including a visit to the library and librarian, Kate Vargo.

Our first day ended with measurements for uniforms – white pants for the men, white skirts for the women, with blue tops for both sexes and white lab coats. I was at the back of the line, waiting to go into the back classroom where people were being measured. While standing on line, the only thing I could think of is, "All of these young women and men standing here, waiting to get their form-fit bodies measured and here I am a portly 35 year-old thinking one wrong move in these "tidy whities" and I'm going to need safety-pins.

Waiting on line, the last thing I remember saying to myself, I might have even mentioned it to the person standing behind me, was "If they make me wear a nurse's cap, how will I pin it to my bald head?"

Standing behind me in line was a very pretty young woman in her early 20s, short blonde hair and very attractive. I asked her name. She said, "I'm Doreen Stetz, how are ya?"

"Well to tell you the truth, Doreen, I'm feeling a little uncomfortable. Looking around on this line, I feel like I'm everybody's grandfather."

She said, "I'm not feeling too comfortable myself. I'm really not into getting my ass measured for uniforms."

I cracked up. I liked Doreen right away and wanted to know more about her.

"What do you have to worry about?" I chimed in. "What are you a size 2?"

"No actually, I'm a 6 or 8, and if they say anything, I'll just give them the finger," she said.

Then she flipped the bird, only I noticed her finger had been partially amputated. That immediately made me feel comfortable talking to her and I thought, we could have some fun here.

"You know Doreen, they said earlier that we need to buddy up and find a study partner," I told her. "I don't know anyone else here, would you like to be my study partner? You make me laugh!"

"Sure," she said. "That sounds fun."

After having my measurements screamed out for everyone to hear, I went home, opened my textbook and once again felt like I'll never get through this. Chapter one, "The 'Fun'damentals of Nursing" didn't look like fun to me.

I could barely sleep that night. The next morning, I got to school and headed downstairs to the Skills Lab, which turned out to be the darkest and dingiest room you could imagine. The practice mannequins had limbs missing. The equipment was old, sub-standard and out of date. And for a class of 75 students to be crammed into that tiny lab room, it was hardly conducive to learning. I remember having to elbow my way to the front of the class to see what the instructor was showing us.

I'm a visual learner. I can't pick up a book, read it and do it. Like my 16 years on the railroad, I had to be the apprentice before I can be the teacher. So it was extremely important that I see the instructor demonstrate the procedures. Then when I read about the procedure, I can picture it in my mind and understand it more clearly.

I went home that Friday after the first week of school and told Bob, "I think I made a big mistake." Bob's response was very typical of him, he was stern but yet supportive saying, and "I know you will make a fantastic nurse, imagine the possibilities and follow your dreams."

I knew he was right, but still I couldn't help think that nursing school was turning out to be more of a nightmare than a dream. I don't expect anyone but a Nurse to understand why I was feeling that way. I thought of Dawn and how she said she would help and I sought her out at school the following Monday.

Dawn saw me and hugged me so tight, and said "Dominick so good to see you, I have so much stuff for you from my freshman year that will help you."

I didn't even have to ask Dawn for help, she already planned it and her support of my success was critical to my getting through the tough times. I now knew an upper classman or should I say upper class-woman?

It took two weeks for the uniforms to arrive and it took about that long for me to adjust to this new lifestyle, which was completely different from everything I had known or experienced.

I took my uniform home, tried it on again, looked in the mirror and visualized myself on graduation day. The feeling of accomplishment had already been there. I felt accomplished just getting to this point. I didn't really know what I was in for, but I was excited to begin a new journey. It sure was a different feeling than that of working on the railroad.

I felt like Dorothy when she landed in Oz and thought she was home free, but didn't know she was going to have to bring that witch's broom back to the Wizard first. I was in school, starting my new journey, doing the best I could, unaware of how many witches' brooms I would soon collect in order to be home free, all of this for an R.N. after my name?

During those first two weeks, we were on a schedule: Fundamentals of Nursing, Monday through Friday, 8 am-to-1 pm with one 15-minute break. And then Saint Peter's College in Jersey City three days a week for required courses in the Sciences. We had to earn 81 credits to graduate, my goodness that seemed like a lot to me.

When I started nursing school, I didn't have a clue as to how difficult it was going to be to get through the schooling part of it. I kind of thought being a nurse won't be a problem. They say, once you get past the poop, piss and the puke you've got it made. Not necessarily. You can take care of people; you can be the most tender, caring, loving person in the clinical setting. You can bring someone from diagnosis to death with total dignity and be absolutely superb at what you do, that people will ask for you to be their caretaker.

But if you can't pass those nursing exams, you can't be a Registered Nurse.

Aside from nursing courses I had to complete the following required courses: English, Pharmacology, Sociology, Psychology, Anatomy and Physiology I & II, Microbiology and Chemistry. Each class was two hours. Afternoons were spent at Saint Peter's College or in one of the school classrooms studying.

We had to get through September and October, before we started clinical rotations, which was when we would be working with patients. We had to learn the basics, make a bed, clean a patient, brush their teeth, comb their hair, dress them, get them out of bed and into a chair – all of these are basic nursing interventions. It is what the Certified Nursing Assistants (CNAs) do.

We learned all of these interventions by watching videos and working in that cramped Skills Lab. We also practiced on one another, which in our study group was always our fun learning time.

One of the mannequins had a arm that was detached so when I was in the hospital bed portraying a patient for class, I put the mannequin's arm between my legs as if I had three and when Doreen pulled the sheets down to do the assessment, she screamed and jumped ten feet in the air.

We were always doing silly things like that. The teachers didn't seem to mind. This wasn't a formal class; it was just practice time. Instructors would look at us, shake their heads and look away. In some ways I think we helped lighten their day. As long as you got it right in skills testing, they didn't care how you went from Point "A" to Point "B".

There was a lot of traveling back and forth between Christ Hospital School of Nursing and St. Peter's College. I could fit three people in my car and they were always Winston, Doreen and Maria; we were always together. – Our version of *The Mod Squad*.

In the first semester I don't think I ever scored a 90% on a nursing exam.

Even though it had been 16 years since I had been in high school, I did very well in science, math, English, anatomy and physiology and microbiology, scoring 'As', 'Bs' and 'B-plusses.' The hands-on stuff came easy for me like setting up IV pumps, giving injections; it was like I belonged there. There was a huge difference between the tests at Saint Peter's and nursing school exams. And now clinical rotations would be starting.

For my first clinical rotation, my instructor was Ms. Emily Marcelo. This rotation was easy for me; it involved bed-making, monitoring blood pressure, communication – sort of like hanging out with your patient to make them feel good. Nurses assigned to the units did most of the real nursing interventions.

A couple of weeks doing clinical rotations, something curious occurred. Pre-clinical assignments were given out the afternoon before our clinical rotations and a female student had been assigned a gay male patient with AIDS. When the Nurse read the chart in the pre-clinic assignment, she gave the student a different patient. The instructors were never present for pre-clinical but they would leave our patient assignments with the charge nurse in our assigned unit.

When the morning nursing staff found out that this young lady was assigned an AIDS patient she was taken off that assignment and the instructor reassigned her a new patient. This did not seem to be a big deal to anyone else but it put me in a panic.

# My Journey as an AIDS Nurse

My sole intention to attend nursing school was to become an AIDS Nurse. And now I find out that there's a rule that students are not allowed to care for patients with HIV/AIDS? How could I possibly specialize in AIDS Care if I can't learn how to care for AIDS patients? What if I have to go through three years of nursing school never to experience caring for a person living with AIDS? Could this derail my plan to become an AIDS Nurse?

I could not sit back and let this happen so the activist in me came out in a big way. I went to Mr. Hebert and filed a grievance, which was a formal process for a nursing student if they thought they were being treated unfairly.

The next day I was called out of Skills Lab to report to Mr. Hebert's office. And as I walked down the dark green hallway, past the photos of all the graduating classes with nurses in their white uniforms, I thought to myself, "Oh my God, I blew it already."

I sat in the outer office and waited. A few minutes later, Mr. Hebert came out, shook my hand ushered me into his private office and closed the door. "Dominick, tell me what is the problem," he said.

"Mr. Hebert, I came to Christ Hospital School of Nursing not only to be a Registered Nurse, but to specialize in AIDS Care. But how can I do that if I'm not allowed to work with patients who have HIV/AIDS?"

"Dominick, I understand your concerns, but we have rules here and that rule has been in place since 1981 to protect our students. We would be extremely negligent if we allowed a student who has no experience working with an AIDS patient to handle an AIDS patient. One mistake could be deadly."

"I understand all that Mr. Hebert, but isn't this a school for nursing? How else am I going to learn? Besides, don't you think that rule is outdated? Back in 1981, we didn't know what we know

now. Times have changed. The rule was valid, back then, I suppose, because no one really knew enough about AIDS or GRID as it was called back in the beginning. But this is 1991. Isn't it time to change the rule?"

I was not going to back down from this. As it turned out Mr. Hebert consulted with Miss Fasano and they took it to the hospital's Board of Directors.

A few days later, Mr. Hebert called me back into his office. He was there with Ms. Marcelo, my clinical instructor and also one of the school's best teachers.

"Dominick, I met with Ms. Fasano, our Director of Nursing and we both met with the Board of Directors at Christ Hospital School of Nursing. We brought up your request to change the rule regarding student nurses and AIDS care and after much discussion, the Board agreed to change the rule. Now, if a student nurse chooses to accept a patient who has HIV/AIDS, they may care for that patient. But if a student is not comfortable caring for a person living with HIV/AIDS, that student also has the right to refuse and get a new assignment."

Well, the activist in me came out again. "If a student nurse does not want to care for a person living with AIDS then perhaps they should go to school for something else," I said.

I could tell by the grin on Ms. Marcelo's face that she totally agreed with me, but Mr. Hebert just calmly said, "I am sure this will change down the line but let's just be happy with this first step for now."

Emily Marcelo pulled me aside afterwards and said, "You keep fighting Dominick, and you will be a leader in this profession."

Those words gave me the drive and the will to succeed.

The very next week, Ms. Marcelo assigned me to the care of Mr. Green, an African-American man in his late 30s early 40s.

Mr. Green was very sick in end-stage AIDS and needed a lot of nursing care.

I went to the hospital chapel before the clinical day started as I did before each clinical rotation and before every exam. My prayer was to help Mr. Green to the best of my ability and give him comfort as he was obviously in pain and unable to get out of bed.

One of the interventions for Mr. Green that day was to remove the old bandages from his feet and replace them with new ones after doing wound care to his heels, which had Stage 3 ulcerations.

As I was taught in class, I had to first do Mr. Green's morning care. He was soiled, so I cleaned him up – just as I did seven months ago for my dear friend Frankie. I kept talking to Mr. Green as I worked although I don't think he was able to understand too much. But we were alone and I just knew I had a lot of work to do removing soiled linens, making an occupied bed and then bandaging his feet.

For a very brief moment I thought "will I ever get through this today" but that feeling passed quickly. I read the treatment order at least three times, gathered my supplies, went back into his room, washed my hands and went to work. As I cut off the old gauze bandages, I visualized myself doing tasks every day of my life. I loved what I was doing at that moment. I was not nervous or frightened in any way. I did that job with all the love and compassion I had inside of me.

Afterwards, I looked at Mr. Green and he did not seem to be in any distress although I was getting little or no response from him. I rolled up a thin throw blanket, what we call a "trochanter roll" (I have no idea why they call it that,) and placed it under his ankles to keep the heels of his feet from touching the bed linens thus giving them a chance to heal.

I finished up, washed my hands again and went to the nurses' station to document what I had done. Nursing documentation is critical and the importance is stressed over and over in nursing school. "If it was not documented, it was not done"

While Mr. Green rested, I wrote everything I did in his chart. I was so focused I didn't see Dr. Len Denbleyker walk up to the Nurses' Station. He is a very handsome podiatrist and all of the female nurses swoon over him.

In the back of my head I can hear "Yes Doctor. No Doctor. Anything you say Doctor."

I looked up just as he was walking away. I think my jaw dropped, not just because he was a hottie, but also because he was headed straight for Mr. Green's room. There had been a podiatry consult written and he was going in to look at the heels of Mr. Green's feet.

I thought I was going to die on the spot. That was the only time I felt nervous. Five minutes later he came out of the room, walked back to the nurses' station.

"Who wrapped Mr. Green's feet?" His voice was loud and deep.

"He was assigned to the student today," Ginny, the charge nurse said. "Is there a problem?"

I really liked Ginny. She had total control over everything that was going on in her unit and took no guff from anyone, not even the doctors – especially not the doctors.

Dr. Denbleyker said, "No, I just wanted to say that that is the best foot wrapping job I have ever seen. Who's the student?"

"Dominick over there at the desk," she said.

He walked over to me and extended his hand. "Thanks, Dominick, you saved me a lot of time today." I was speechless as we shook hands.

This is the reason why you have to put love, care and compassion into everything you do for all of your patients all of the time. You never know when you will run into someone important or who is watching your every move.

Dr. Denbleyker asked me if I wanted a job at his office as a nurse when I graduate. I thanked him and said "No thanks. If I ever get out of here I'm going to be an AIDS Nurse."

In the nursing courses, we had four 50-question tests throughout the semester, one a month. And the week after the fourth test, we had a final exam of 100 questions. So, here's how it breaks down. Each of the four tests counts as 15 percent of the grade and the final exam counts as 30 percent of your grade and then 10 percent is for special assignments, like clinical, oral presentations, essays and one quiz in nursing assessment. I did relatively well, never getting higher than a 90 on a test; my highest was 88, and holding my own. Throughout the semester I scored in the low to mid 80s.

Even though I was getting good scores I was nervous about the final exam. We were all nervous about the nursing exams. In a nursing exam, there are two correct answers for every question and one answer is more correct than the other so it makes it twice as difficult. They do that to build your critical thinking skills.

You have to know what you would do first and then second. In other words, you have to be able to think on your feet. I knew I was going to do okay. What I wanted to do was get an exceptional grade for the final, not just passing. The exam was so hard – 100 questions that had to be completed in two hours. All our instructors walked around to make sure there was no cheating. It was intense.

I got my test score back pretty quickly; they posted the results on the student bulletin board.

I scored a 74 on the final, which brought my average for the semister to an 82, which was passing. (70% was passing.) I was happy I got through it.

My study group friends Winston, Doreen and Maria also passed. We saw each other in the hallway and hugged. I called Bob to tell him my good news; and we planned to celebrate that night.

# Emotional Roller Coaster

I no sooner had hung up with Bob when I got a call from Virginia that Red was gravely ill and that I should come down right away and say my goodbyes. I got in my car and started driving down to Ocean Grove. I can't even tell you how many things were going through my head. I was so happy that I passed the first semester, but I was also feeling like I was on an emotional roller coaster. My first railroad mentor was dying. In order to dispel the thoughts bouncing in my head, I turned on the radio and the song; "Wind Beneath My Wings" was playing. I had to pull over on the shoulder of the Parkway. I just couldn't drive anymore. And then the thoughts started racing again. I needed to get down there for Virginia. I needed to get down there to see Red one more time.

When I got to Virginia's, she wept as she hugged me. I just said to myself, "Get tough. Because there's more of this in your future." So I pulled myself together to be strong for her, but I was dying inside of my own body having to bear this grief just as I had so many times already when one of my friends died from AIDS. I can hear my father in my head saying, "Men don't cry."

We went directly to Jersey Shore Medical Center where I could say my final goodbyes to Red Kimball. I drove Virginia home. There was nothing more we could do. I stayed with

Virginia for most of the day, we talked, we laughed, we cried. She knew I needed to go home so I could celebrate the end of my first semester with Bob. Virginia told me she would call me as soon as she heard from the hospital.

When I returned home I was torn apart with grief but Bob and I decided that I needed to celebrate my accomplishment – I had passed my first semester. We toasted my accomplishment, and we toasted Red Kimball also for the roll he played in my life, and for never judging me for being gay. It was plain and simple Red loved me and accepted me just the way I am.

The next morning, a Saturday, the phone rang. It was Virginia telling me that Red had died during the night. I was not shocked but I was devastated. Why should I bother being a nurse when everyone dies anyway? Do I really want this life? Can I go through this again and again? I was torturing myself, until Virginia said to me, "Walter will be watching you as you go through school. He knows you will be a fine nurse."

# 1992
# Still in the game

Coming back to school after nearly a month off was very difficult. I wasn't even sure if I really wanted to continue. We started out with 75 students in our first semester and now there were 57 starting our second semester; 18 people didn't come back.

We started classes on a Tuesday and the first lecture was a lesson we would need to learn and carry with us the rest of our lives. It was about critical thinking, a term used by all nurses every day.

The first week back my classmates gave me something to think about, they nominated me for class president probably because I was the oldest male nursing student in class. It could also have been because they knew I was an AIDS activist and saw me in action the first semester when I fought to change the rule regarding students caring for AIDS patients. I decided to step up as I usually do and was elected.

While I was really good at fundraising and helping to put the class yearbook together it became increasingly difficult for me to concentrate on my studies. I began to fail tests and quizzes. I knew I had to step up my game; my priority was becoming a nurse, not class president.

The clinical rotation in my second semester came easy to me. I excelled in clinical practice and also my courses at St. Peter's College. Now, if I could only pass these nursing exams my life would be so much better. With school taking up every minute of my day and weekends too, I rarely had a chance to see friends. I had to give up my post as vice president of the Garden State Gay Bowling Organization (GSGBO) and I would only sub at bowling because Wednesdays and Thursdays were my mornings for clinical rotation and I had to be at the hospital by 6:30 am for rounds. My life became school, funerals, and the occasional party.

This was also the semester that we began our 12-week segments for the three required nursing specialties: pediatrics, OB-GYN and psychiatric nursing. There were 19 of us in each rotation; and I was assigned pediatrics with Ms. DeCena as my instructor.

Pediatrics was fun but I just could not get the hang of it. I passed all of my pediatrics exams but playing with kids was not why I wanted to be a nurse. Thank God the twelve weeks went quickly. I did well in pediatrics and to tell you the truth I had fun playing with and caring for the kids. They made me laugh, have fun, and see nursing with a more light-hearted spirit, something I would not have accomplished without my pediatric rotation.

In Sociology class we learned that Maslow described self-actualization as the desire for one to see oneself in his fullest potential. I kept thinking I would never be able to say I was "self actualized" even after reading the definitions over and over – I was still doubting myself.

That semester, my English teacher Professor Corless gave me the drive to keep trying. I told her about my failing grades in the nursing courses and she said, "You will pass Dominick, and you will be a great nurse."

From that point on I passed every test that semester. The first semester my average was in the 80s and this semester I passed in the mid 70s.

In the middle of May, right before my final two tests, Bob graduated from Stern's School of Business at NYU with an MBA and began studying for the CPA exam. School seemed to come easy for Bob. He would read and study and just had the knack to remember everything.

My study group made up mock nursing tests to practice before the real test and when Bob would help me study he would take those tests and get a better grade than I did. He would show me why I got the answer wrong. Had it not been for Bob's help, I would not be a Nurse today.

# Place your bets

After my freshman year, I took a summer job as a nursing assistant at South Amboy Memorial Hospital working the 11 pm-to-7 am shift. My first night at South Amboy turned out to be the night that would either make or break my career as a nurse. I got there early and listened to the shift report from the 3-to-11 shift nurses.

There was one RN, Marylou, and one LPN, Peggy, and I was their assistant. My first assignment was to do vital signs on every patient; there were 20 patients in ten rooms. In order for the nurses to be able to perform their duties I would have to write down the blood pressure reading and turn it in to the Nurse in a timely manner. This was not supposed to be a difficult task. It was almost midnight so I had to be as quiet as possible and I could not turn lights on in the rooms so the only light I had was the light from the hallway.

I went into the first room and took the vital signs of the man in bed "A" near the door. All was good so far, so I wrote down the vitals on my pad and went to bed "B". I was in full swing, or so I thought. As I exited that first room into the hallway both nurses were hysterical laughing at me. What did I do? What was the joke?

I looked down and saw two brown stripes across my white uniform. The sick man in bed "B" had smeared his side-rails with poop and I leaned into the side-rails to take his blood pressure. Fortunately, the Nurses had extra scrubs and I put on the clean scrubs and washed myself up and moved on with my work. I then had to clean him and the side rails and do 18 more blood pressures.

In Room 9, there was a woman in the bed near the window, and when I took her blood pressure it seemed really low, and her breathing was not right. I did not know what was wrong, but when I took her wrist to take her pulse it was cold as ice and I had difficulty finding a pulse. This did not seem good to me, but I was just a first-year nursing student, so I went to the nursing station and reported my findings to the LPN.

I didn't realize it then, but I was using my critical thinking skills. She called for the RN and they ran into the room. I followed behind. These nurses seemed to know just what to do. I ran for extra blankets and watched as they raised the bed up a little.

It was 5 am when the woman died. I knew from school that when someone dies in the hospital the family has to be called and then the nursing staff has to do post-mortem care and wrap the body. The family members came up just before she took her last breath and did have a chance to say good-bye. Since I had not done my Psych rotation, I did not realize the significance of that at that time.

Getting the family there to transition the patient from life to death is one of the most important duties of a nurse. We were on the fourth floor and everyone was crying. That made me feel like I was at the funeral of a person I didn't even know. By 8:30 we all left and I could barely keep my eyes open for the 40-minute drive back home.

Before I left one of the nurses asked me, "Are we going to see you tonight?" I was so delirious from the long night that I didn't even realize I had to do this again in less than 16 hours. I did come back that night and learned that Marylou and Peggy had made a bet on me, one thought I would end my nursing career after my first night and the other said I'll be back. Marylou won the bet and I won favor that night of two really terrific nurses.

## Putting me to the testes

The fall semester of my second year as a student nurse was wonderful compared to my first year. I even took a part-time job at Christ Hospital on the Psychiatric Unit as a Psychiatric Technician. I loved that job and learned so much from the staff.

Meanwhile, back at school, I had two very special patients in my clinical rotation. My first patient was a 40-year-old man, Jose. I was reading his chart, which stated that he was being tested for testicular cancer. I went down to the skills lab, got the testicular model, brought it over the hospital and said to him, "This is the model of the testicles. To learn how to find lumps, you can practice with this then you will know how to check yourself. It's the same way we teach a woman to examine her breasts for lumps."

I had him try it on the model first. I put the rocks in and then he felt them as I instructed him to. Then he examined his own testicles, and said, "I think there's a lump. I feel a lump in my testicle." "Do you want me to get the doctor to confirm it?" I asked?

He said, "No, I want you to do it."

This told me he was comfortable with my teaching method to allow me to check him. It turns out, I did not find a lump in his testicle, the charge nurse verified my findings and the staff commended me. It was a good find.

After all the relevant tests were completed, he was diagnosed with Epididymitis, a bacterial infection. He wanted to know if, after the treatment, would he be able to have full sexual function again without pain. We told him 'yes' and he was a happy man. He said to me, "If it wasn't for you. I would have lost my mind."

In nursing school, we were taught to do complete assessments, first the demographic information like where do you live; how many children do you have? These are the easy questions and most people won't refuse to give you their demographics.

Then it's on to family history. Most patients know their family and those who do not; well we just can't put down information they can't give you. Communication about mental health history is a little more difficult. The nurse knows to work from the more global questions to the more specific questions. It is not easy to ask a person if they ever had suicide ideation, because you never know what will come out of it. Still it has to be done in order to have a complete assessment.

Last, sitting with a patient and getting their sexual history, their most private and intimate health concerns, is not easy for some people to do. For me to ask someone "Have you ever had unprotected sex? Are you high risk for this illness or that illness" is easy. You do a head to toe assessment and when you get to the middle of the body you have to talk about the private parts. Some practitioners shy away from it. Even today, I read hospital charts where it says "penis, vagina, rectum or breasts – and you see next to it "assessment-deferred," which means the patient refused to give the information. Sometimes, I think it's the doctor who means to say, "I did not care to go there."

One of the reasons why AIDS is still prevalent is because many health care professionals defer examination of the genitalia, and thus never getting an accurate sexual history. Granted it is difficult to talk about, but how many times does a person have to leave a doctor's office or a hospital knowing that something's wrong and never being asked about it. If that person does have AIDS, by the time they figure it out, it could be too late.

## Here Comes the Son

My next patient was a woman diagnosed with cancer and just days left to live. Four of her children were with her. She was being put on palliative care. She rarely spoke.

I had to clean her and change her linens. I knew it was her time, but she was holding on for some reason. I said to the family, "Go get a cup of coffee and come back and allow me to do her morning care and talk to her."

"She doesn't talk to us, I don't think she'll talk to you," her son said.

The DNR order (Do Not Resuscitate), and the DNI order (Do Not Intubate) were in place and everyone knew she was nearing the end. The hospital social worker spoke to the family about hospice care.

Meanwhile, I felt she was holding on to something. Part of my job as a nurse was to communicate with her. Knowing communication was difficult for her, I had to utilize my skills in non-verbal communication. I looked directly at her and said: "I know it may be difficult for you to respond to my questions, but we can communicate with our eyes. A while back you mentioned your son. Is there another son that you were speaking of who is not here today?"

She nodded "yes".

"Has he visited you?"

The look in her eyes told me he had not. I talked a little more about my own family, and mentioned that we were a family of five siblings as well. The questions asked were somewhat global and as I learned in Nursing 101, we needed to work from global to specific. When I reached the specific, I gathered that her youngest son had never visited her and was probably in denial about her impending death.

When her four other children returned from the cafeteria, I spoke with her son. I told him what she had implied in our non-verbal communication.

"She must be waiting for my younger brother.," he said to me. I asked him, "Is there any way you can get him to visit her? She needs to see him."

The next morning, I went up to the Clinical Unit Nurses' Station prior to going to class to ask how my patient was doing. They told me she died at 4 am.

"Did she get to see her youngest son?" I asked.

The Nurse at the station said some family members are still in the room. I went there and saw her son gathering her cards, robe, slippers, and the clothes she wore when she was admitted.

"Thank you," he said.

"Did she get to see your brother?"

"Yes. He came in about 11 pm. We left him alone with her. And he left about midnight. That was all he could take. We got called back to the hospital around 3 am and we stayed with her until she passed."

Some people let go when they're ready and God was ready for her and she wasn't letting go until she saw her youngest son. I thought about this and I realized it's the miracle of life into death.

# Big Boys Don't Cry

I was now in my second required rotation, OB-GYN, and was learning things about the female anatomy that I never knew.

The strange thing is that of the three specialties OB-GYN was the most rewarding. Two of my female patients that semester actually wrote letters to the hospital complimenting the post-partum care they received from their male student nurse. These were the same two patients who, in the beginning, did not want a male nurse to care for them. After I talked to them, they agreed to allow me to be their nurse. If that didn't work, I would then have to go in there, snap my fingers and say, "Girls, I'm gay, get over it!" Instead, I told them they had no choice in the matter and I assured them I would maintain the utmost professionalism. If they still did not allow me to be their nurse, I would not have passed that rotation.

The most memorable moment that term was when eight of the students witnessed the natural birth of a baby girl – including me. The next day in lecture our instructor Dorothy Roseborrough mentioned we saw the miracle of childbirth and went on to say "...and Dominick was the only one who cried"

I was mortified!

Between classes at Saint Peter's College, I was sitting with some of my classmates when this young kid, at least ten years my junior, walked up to me and asked, "Is your name Dominick Varsalone?"

"Yes."

"Do you remember me?" he asked.

"I'm sorry I don't," I said.

"You were my coach in Little League," he said.

I immediately flashed back to those days when I was a married man, working for the railroad and coaching a Little League team at Lincoln Park in Jersey City. I then recognized who he was.

My name is Billy," he said.

I remembered him as a not-so-great baseball player, but I never gave up on him. He was a good kid and I liked him and his dad, too. Billy played every single game and the game that I recall was when he got his first base hit and brought in the winning run. Everybody on the team lifted him up, like a scene in the movie *Bad News Bears*, where the player least likely to get a hit gets his chance to be the hero.

Billy's dad would tell me that even though our team didn't win the championship or have many wins, he considered me a great coach because I gave everybody an equal chance. For Billy to remember me 10 years later was a real boost to my confidence.

"What are you doing at Saint Peter's College?" Billy asked. "Don't you work on the railroad anymore?"

Billy remembered I used to come to practice straight from the South Kearny Railroad Yard where I worked.

"I almost didn't recognize you without your coveralls." he said.

"No, I'm going to nursing school now," I told him. "No more coveralls for me."

## Grandma Nightingale

One of my classmates, Natasha, was the oldest woman in our class, and since I was the oldest man, the younger students referred to us as "Grandma" and "Grandpa".

Natasha was a Russian immigrant who was a physician in Russia. She was very smart, but she could not understand the English expressions we used. American slang was not in her dictionary.

Natasha taught herself how to speak English and she did a great job. Still, she had a very thick Russian accent and most people could not understand her. Because she was a doctor, she was very helpful to the students, including me. She taught us nursing at the cellular level, some of the real concepts of why things have to be the way they are with some illnesses and diseases. I, in turn, helped her with American slang.

One day, we were sitting in anatomy and physiology class and the professor was talking to us about illnesses of the brain. He explained that 60 percent of the brain is white matter and 40 percent of the brain is gray matter. With inactivity, the gray matter begins to soften and turns gelatinous.

"The gray matter in your brain will turn to goop," he said.

43

All I could hear behind me was Natasha flipping through the pages of her dictionary, looking for "goop." I suddenly went flying forward when Natalia whacked me on the right shoulder. "What is this goop?" she shouts out in frustration. "It's like jelly or ice cream," I whispered. She finally got it.

Doreen, Natasha, Winston, Maria and I came from different cultures and had different religious beliefs and sexual orientations, but we worked well as a study group because different perspectives were brought into our discussions. Many of our study group meetings were held at my home. I would make meatball surprise and everybody loved it. Cooking was my biggest contribution to the group, not academics.

# Boys to Men

During the fall semester of my second year of nursing school, on November 18, Pasquale, my childhood best friend, a man I loved like a brother, died of AIDS. This loss really knocked the wind out of my sails and caused me to withdraw somewhat. A month later I was taking my final exam, and I wasn't prepared. It was the only final in three years of nursing school that I failed, but thank God my average was high enough to keep my grade above 70. There is no logical reason why I failed. I was doing well in school, but the loss of Pasquale was life altering. I felt vulnerable and afraid.

Pasquale's wife, Anna, who we went to high school with, was happy to see me at his funeral. We had lost contact after high school and I think they knew I had come out of the closet since then. Maybe he knew all along I was gay and loved me and protected me anyway. That's the way I want to look at it. I never did have the guts to tell anyone that Pasquale was my first man-crush but of course I had suppressed that, like so many other secrets.

After Pasquale died, the rest of my school year was a blur. My average that semester was 78. I continued to work on the Psych Unit to help pay the bills and to learn as much about psychiatric nursing as possible because my final specialty rotation was coming up next. My teacher would be Ms. S, and she looked like a tough one.

# 1993
# Miss Diagnosed

It was back to school and for the first two weeks everything was going well, and my class got into the swing of things easily. After three semesters, we were old pro Nursing Students. The first person I see was, Professor Coreless. I thanked her for her words of encouragement from the last two semesters. Professor Coreless was very professional and she was not an automatic hugger. She did ask me, however, if she could give me a hug and of course I said, yes. I am Italian after all and we know how to hug.

On our first day back, Ms. S. gave a lecture and I liked her right away. She had a tough way about her like many of the Psych Nurses on 5 East, but in order to be a great Psych Nurse you have to be tough. You have to show people with mental illness that you are not afraid to help them, especially when they are off their medications or acting out. For many nursing students this can be a very frightening experience.

Ms. S. taught us a great deal in the first few weeks and then we would do our clinical rotations. I was so happy to have a tremendous advantage going into this rotation and I thought I would sail through it. We had our first exam after week three and I got a 68. I was so upset because I really thought I knew the terminology and I was certain that I knew how to answer the critical thinking questions. I had been not only thinking about psych nursing I was working at the Psych Unit.

At the time, I learned an important lesson that would carry me through nursing school and the rest of my nursing career. Every nursing student should know before they start that just because a Nurse working on the unit does a particular intervention a certain way does not mean it is the correct way, or the right answer to a question on a test. I learned this the hard way.

I think Ms. S was disappointed in me because she expected me to get the highest grade in the class on that first test because of my experience in the Psych unit. I was sorry I disappointed her but more so, I was terrified that this would be the term that would make me the next student to fail out.

In lecture the following week, we were talking about the DSM (Diagnostic and Statistical Manual) books that housed the rules and regulations of Psychiatric Mental Health. Ms. S seemed especially tough on me that day which I thought was because of my test score. We were on the topic of homosexuality, and how it was considered a mental illness with a diagnosis in previous DSMs.

Everyone in the class knew I was gay and no one had an issue with it. Unlike the harassment I had endured while working on the railroad, none of my classmates knew what had happened to me because I didn't tell anyone. I just wanted to forget the past and move on with my life.

I thought I was doing that until this lecture when Ms. S. announced to the whole class that I was "mentally ill" for being gay. I don't think she meant to call me out that way – or did she? Nurses in psychiatric care should be tough, but not mean-spirited. I only know that the entire class laughed at me and I lost it. I yelled out a few choice words and excused myself from the rest of the lecture.

She then told the class that I did not have what it takes to be a nurse if I can't take a little criticism. I went outside for a minute to think about what I was going to do next. I was so upset I could hardly breathe. No one came out to check on me, or ask if I was all right. I then decided to go to Mr. Hebert. I told him I could not allow Ms. S to treat me that way and I would not continue to go to her class and have her harass me like my managers at South Kearny Railway. Mr. Hebert excused me for the rest of the day and said he would handle it. I came to school the next day and was told by Mrs. Killman, the House Mother to report directly to Director of Nursing Ms. Fasano's office, and was met there by Ms. Fasano and Mr. Hebert.

I thought they were going to expel me. Instead I was told that Ms. S would be giving her notice in two weeks and they asked if I would be able to take her class for two weeks until a substitute teacher could be found. I told them I would agree to that.

The students in my class loved her and they all rebelled against me. Once again I was feeling miserable about being gay and the only person in my class who stood by me through it all was Doreen. She was so upset, and kept telling me "it will be all right."

Doreen was right. After a few weeks, we had a new teacher and while most everyone in my class stopped talking to me, I was doing much better on my exams. With Ms. P. as our new instructor, I passed every one of the next three exams and got a terrific grade on the final. Psych nursing was my most successful rotation. In addition, when I took the Psych National League of Nursing exam, I scored in the 95 percentile.

# Up, Up and Away

I met Matt and Barry through my very special friend, Teresa who I met at a rehearsal for "Take Off with U.S.", a musical revue put on by a new theater troupe in Jersey City. We got to know each other at the diner we would go to after rehearsals. She was a social worker with plans to be a lawyer, and I liked her because she was very witty and smart, and I think she was the best friend I could have had at that time in my life. I was still at a crossroads with my sexuality, and I would confide in Teresa and she would offer me great advice. Always did.

At the end of the summer of '81, I had just returned from a Gay Softball Tournament in Toronto, and when I invited Teresa over to catch up, I opened the door and she was standing there with a suitcase in her hand.

"You planning to stay a while?" I joked. She started to cry and told me she was going through a rough patch at home. I invited Teresa to stay with me for as long as she needed, and in an instant I had a roommate.

We would throw weekend dinner parties and I soon learned Teresa had more gay friends than I did, like Matt and Barry who were flight attendants for a major airline. It's not every day you meet a couple that met 30,000 feet in the air. They were a perfect match; just like Bob and me.

Matt had been in and out of the hospital several times with all kinds of AIDS-related complications. He told Barry that on his 30th birthday he was going to stop taking his medications, give up the fight, and let God take over from there. It was up to Barry to insist Matt fight back or support Matt's decision to give up. Barry stood by Matt and invited his family to their Greenwich Village apartment to let them know Matt's decision.

About half of Matt's family agreed that it should be done just the way Matt wanted it to be done and the other half was resistant. Bob and I decided to support Matt's decision and Matt signed the DNR, came home from the hospital and remained home without any AIDS medications. The only thing he insisted on was a morphine drip to not feel any pain.

Bob and I were back and forth to Matt and Barry's apartment as often as possible to help out. I brought my stethoscope and my medical bag each time we went. Someone needed to be there for Barry who was a wonderful spouse to Matt and a great friend to us.

The next time the phone rang, it was Rich. Ben, his partner of several years, was in Christ Hospital clinging to life. Every day I went to school, I stopped and saw Ben. Then I would go home to eat and run over to New York City to see Matt. Bob would sometimes go after work and meet me there. I would come home at 9 or 10 pm, prepare for my lessons at school and do it all over the next day.

On March 11, I had stopped in to see Ben after school while outside snow was falling hard. The weather forecasters were predicting 'The Storm of the Century,' and nurses could not make it into work, so when I arrived, no one on staff was available to take care of Ben who had soiled himself. So, I took it upon myself to go to the clean linen room and get the needed supplies. I gave him a bed bath, cleaned and dried him off, shaved his face and put him in a fresh gown. I then changed the bed linens. I remembered a little trick that a nursing assistant taught me. I powdered the sheets with baby powder, even though it wasn't part of our instruction at nursing school.

I fluffed Ben's pillow and raised the head of his bed so he could breathe a little easier. I left for home and by the time I got there several inches of snow had fallen. When I woke up Friday, school had been canceled. The storm was really bad and no one could go anywhere or do anything except shovel snow. I shoveled several times that day. Bob stayed home from work and baked and cooked dinner. The phone rang and it was Rich. He was crying, so I knew Ben had died. I also received a call from Ben's family, thanking me for being there for him, especially the day before he died. I was quickly missing Ben, and still thinking about Matt, how much time would he have left. It was not a happy time for any of us. Matt was off his medication for 17 days, New York and New Jersey were buried in snow. I think they had to hold off on Ben's burial for a little while. The only bright spot at this time was the fact that Bill Clinton was our new president.

After his first 50 days in office President Clinton vowed to increase funding for AIDS research and join the fight against AIDS. We finally had a President that got the point. The following week I was back at school, but going back and forth to New York to visit Matt was still difficult. I came home from school and my phone was ringing. It was Barry telling me Matt's time was near and he wanted me to be there. I called Bob and I met him at Matt and Barry's apartment.  It was exactly one month after Matt's 30th birthday.

Everyone in Matt's family was there, along with some close friends including Bob who arrived just before me. It was so surreal, everyone was sitting in the living room and Matt was lying in bed with the morphine drip running and oxygen flowing. Barry was holding Matt's hand and talking to him and I was on the other side with my stethoscope around my neck.

I was checking Matt's pulse, and taking his blood pressure every half hour. I was watching him breathe, and everything seemed normal. Blood pressure was in the normal range; pulse was 70, respirations 16, and not labored. Suddenly, Matt removed the oxygen mask from his face, sat up in bed and asked Barry to walk him into the living room where everyone was sitting.

I started to sweat because I had never seen this kind of calm before.

Matt stood in the living room and said to everyone, "I am ready to go now, please don't be sad. I love you all, but I am tired and I need to go to sleep now." Then Barry and I put Matt to bed, he winked at me and I left them alone and joined the others.

Barry adjusted the IV and about an hour later asked me to come in and check on Matt. There was no pulse, no blood pressure and no respirations. I was shaking and crying because I had silently pronounced Matt's death. As a Nursing Student I was not allowed to do this by law. So we had to call 911 and the EMS arrived to officially pronounce him dead.

The next morning, I had to be up early for school. With all that was going on with my Psych instructor, and with Ben dying just 11 days prior, and no one to really talk to about it, my first inclination was to get to the chapel, where I had a good cry. I thought I was going to have a breakdown. How can life be so cruel? What could I possibly do in AIDS Care?

We were all there at Matt's wake and funeral, those of us who were left. Matt's family still battled with the why question. Why did he stop taking his medication? Teresa, Bob and I bought a beautiful flower arrangement in the shape of an AIDS ribbon with gold leaf edging, all red carnations. The ribbon across it read "Beloved Friend".

# My Funny Girlfriend

Nursing school does not have to be all work and no play. The funniest times were usually with my dear girlfriend Doreen. I call her girlfriend because she used to call me her best "girlfriend" in nursing school. In our last clinical for Psych nursing, we went to the Ramapo Ridge Psychiatric facility where we spent much of that semester. Doreen always made me laugh, and this day was no exception. All the students in that Psych rotation were attending a support group meeting being given by the social worker. Each student had to sit next to one of the patients and we all had to participate.

The woman patient sitting next to me was experiencing transference – with me. Maybe she thought I was her son or nephew, but she latched onto me like I was someone she loved. She started whispering in my ear.

Sitting directly across from me was a red-faced Doreen who was trying to contain her laughter to the point of almost peeing herself. I kept looking up at Doreen and shrugging my shoulders as if to say, "girlfriend what is your problem?" and "what are you laughing at?"

This went on periodically throughout the group and every time I looked up at Doreen she was still laughing. At the end of the group I asked Doreen what was so funny. It seems the friendly patient talking in my ear had Tardive Dyskinesia, which is the involuntary darting of the tongue in patients who take certain medications for mental health issues.

Doreen was at the perfect angle and told me that as my patient was whispering to me throughout the time in-group it looked as if she was darting her tongue in and out of my ear.

Only Doreen could make nursing school this much fun and it really broke the ice for me because this entire semester was all hard work, and serious business.

As for school, I was really learning what it takes to be a Nurse. My instructors, and the Nurses on the units where I did my clinical rotations, and my dear friends on 5 East, were all terrific. I ended that semester in good shape. I would continue to work on

5 East through the summer until graduation, and I would start my senior year with all my college credits completed. Yes, all 81 credits. I was beginning to see the light at the end of the tunnel.

There were segments of the summer when I wasn't working when I had to visit friends in the hospital or go to another funeral.

## The Ice Bag Cometh

It was now the first day of class and the beginning of senior year. I was elated because Doreen and I had the same clinical rotation at Christ Hospital across the street every Wednesday and Thursday. Our clinical instructor was Rose O'Connor (ROC). She was a no-nonsense instructor who specialized in orthopedics. Doreen and I were a team, and ROC allowed us to work in pairs because traction was sometimes a job for two nurses. Turning patients and setting up traction devices was difficult for one person alone. I had no problem figuring out the devices and ROC expected me to assist the other students in the class who were having difficulties. We were also assigned two or three patients per team, and we had to do all the charting as well.

Two or three care plans were to be turned in by the morning lecture on Friday. God help you if they were not done. My strength was one-to-one care and Doreen knew how to do a care plan, so we made the perfect team.

As usual Doreen made the experience not only fun, but also funny. One of her patients was an older man who had been in traction and bed-bound for quite some time. Doreen and I were in the conference room reading our charts when suddenly Doreen starts laughing. She asked if I would switch patients with her, but would not say why. Of course we were not allowed to switch patients but we could work together, so I asked her what was the problem with this guy? She burst out laughing and said. "Right up your alley; he has edematous balls." She then went on to say, "What the hell am I supposed to do for that?"

"I don't know," I said, "maybe we should read the chart again and see what interventions the previous nurses charted."

The solution was quite easy. Doreen had to chill an IV solution bag and place it under her patient's scrotum for comfort and reduction of swelling. The next day while in the middle of clinic I was in the clean utility room getting some linens to do a bed change. As I opened the door to exit, Doreen pushed me back in the linen closet. "Really, no jokes here, okay?" Doreen was almost in tears from laughing, "I can't do it," she said to me. "I just can't do it!"

"What is wrong with you, girlfriend," I replied. "Snap out of it. You are not being very compassionate here."

Thank God, ROC was not on the unit. As seniors we were supposed to be able to work unsupervised. I told Doreen I would help her out.

When I finished my assignments I went into her patient's room with her and Doreen instructed me to pull up the hospital gown and help her figure out how to place the IV bag under two swollen testes the size of grapefruits. I spoke with Doreen's patient and explained what we were about to do.

"Sir, my name is Dominick and I am Nurse Doreen's colleague. We are about to place a cool IV bag under your scrotum to give you some comfort and relief."

The patient looked at me and shook his head in approval, Doreen and I donned our gloves, and I carefully held up the man's testicles while Doreen carefully placed the IV bag under his scrotum. We were both relieved when the patient let out a very loud, "ah, that feels so good."

## Tragedy Strikes Close to Home

Slightly more than a month had past, and Bob and I received a call from my cousins Bobby and Rosemary. Bobby said, "Hey Cousin, something terrible has happened and we need you and Bob to come to 84 DeKalb Avenue right away."

So, we got in the car and drove to DeKalb Avenue in Jersey City.

When we arrived there was yellow police tape all around her house. We knew this did not look good and from the sound of Bobby's voice, we feared the worse. As we started up the steps, a policeman at her front door yelled, "Hey where do you think you're going?"

"This is my cousin Marge's house," I said, "and her brother Bobby just called me to come over right away."

"Okay," he said, "what are your names?"

"Dominick Varsalone and Robert Buhr" I said. And the officer checked his book and said, "Go in!"

Rosemary saw us, hugged us, and started to cry. "Margie is dead!" she said, "she was murdered!"

I was in shock and so was Bob. Who would want to do this to her? Bobby came over and we hugged "Bobby, what the heck happened?"

"I can't tell you anything until the police speak with you and Bob. They have to question everyone who knew her and had contact with her in the last month."

Bob and I had spent the summer between first and second year nursing school living upstairs from Marge while work was being done on our place. Knowing Bob loved to bake, Marge gave him one of her two rolling pins that had been in the family for many years. We had just had a lunch date with cousin Marge a few weeks before she died.

I couldn't believe Bob and I were called to the scene and questioned by the police about Marge's murder. After answering a few questions we were allowed to talk with Bobby and Rosemary. It was a difficult time for them and I hope our presence gave them some comfort.

I was a nervous wreck during this whole process and I was getting ready for my last two tests in in that semester and also working as many hours as I could on 5 East to help pay the bills. I remember going home isolating myself and crying my eyes out. My cousin was murdered, and life just seemed to be getting more and more crazy as time went on.

The first thing I did when I went to school on Tuesday was head right to ROC's office, which was downstairs across from the skills lab. I told her what had happened to my cousin and that I would need to take some time for the wake and funeral. The school administrators once again were very understanding. We had just had a break for Thanksgiving, and were preparing for the last break before our final six months of school.

# Excessive Thrust

As far as the lectures and exams, ROC was focusing us on the endocrine and skeletal systems. I did well on every test and so did Doreen; it was our best rotation. There was still a lot to learn. Our study group decided to come together at my house again to study for the final. Once again even in the stage of deep grief that I was in, Doreen made me laugh. We all made up cards and questions and one of my card questions was, "New onset Diabetes can cause which of the following symptoms to occur:

A- Hot Flashes
B- Baldness
C- Excessive *thrust*
D- None of the above"

Doreen started laughing when she read the question because I put down thrust instead of thirst. She was making obscene hip thrust movements and screaming "I have diabetes" We all got such a good hearty laugh out of it and then called it quits and had baked ziti and meatballs. For weeks afterwards, Doreen would look at my face and if I did not look happy she would grind her hips and say, "I have diabetes". I would crack up and get back to reality.

# 1994
# Limping to the Finish Line

The last six months of nursing school, were the toughest for me. I had Critical Care with the ICU, CCU instructor Ms. Franne. This final semester we would learn about nursing procedures in the Intensive Care Unit, Critical Care Unit, Operating Room procedures, Emergency Room procedures and Blood Transfusions. Not only were the clinical tasks difficult, the exams were, too.

I ran downstairs after the first exam and saw my grade, 56%.

I cracked and immediately went across the street to the hospital chapel to yell at God. I had to blame someone. I thought I would never recover from that grade and I saw myself going through the entire three years only to fail out at the end. I was so upset that when Bob got home from work I told him I was thinking of just dropping the whole idea of becoming a nurse. He was not happy with me and told me I was being foolish to have done all that work only to give up.

Once again he was right, what else could I say? I cut my hours at work, and I didn't socialize with family or friends. Everyone understood and allowed me to do what I needed to do.

Ms. Franne was a great instructor, as were all the instructors at Christ Hospital School of Nursing. I know I complained about them being strict and regimented about every little detail, but as time went on I understood why they had to be that way.

Ms. Franne was a great teacher especially with ICU and CCU training. She knew everything about ventilators, respirators – I swear she invented the Iron Lung. The IV pumps were constantly lit up; meds were no longer given orally like in previous rotations, because in ICU and CCU most patients could no longer swallow pills. It seemed like every 15 minutes we were performing some type of intervention, like suctioning patients, which was particularly un-nerving for me until I got the hang of it. Soon, I was doing everything almost instinctively, like I had been performing these procedures for years and years. I was enjoying the role I had as a senior class Nursing Student with the exception of one thing: those damn exams, which were kicking my butt.

During OR and ER training, Mrs. Growney, our class advisor, would be right with us watching our every move. The ER was very fast paced at Christ Hospital, as I imagine it is at most hospitals. In OR training, I was about to observe a leg amputation due to diabetes. I knew I would be observing from behind a glass window, that is, until the surgeon noticed the last name on my nametag.

"Varsalone, any relation to Tony Varsalone?" he asked.

"He's my uncle," I said.

"Well then, I want you to assist me in surgery. You can hold the leg while I cut it. Just make sure I am cutting off the correct leg."

"Yes, sir."

"You know why I said correct leg and not right leg?'

"Yes sir, because you will be cutting off the left leg below the knee, not the 'right' leg."

"That is correct," he said. "Would you like to assist?"

"Yes, I would!"

"Scrub up and don't faint into my sterile field," he said.

At the end of the procedure, which seemed like it took all of ten minutes, the surgeon asked me to take the leg to pathology and said, "Good job young man, and tell your Uncle Tony I said hello."

Mrs. Growney asked me to tell my classmates about the experience in post clinical, which I did. I may be the only student, at least that year that actually got to be inside the OR during the rotation.

All I had left to do was a Blood Transfusion. I think this scared me the most. One wrong move and a patient could instantly go into shock and die. At least that is what they told us in class.

# Three

## 1996
## Reflections of the Way Life Used to Be...

When I enter James' room at Broadway House, he is sitting on the edge of the bed staring down at his hands. He looks about 50, but the chart I'm holding says he's 32. It's easy to see he was handsome back in the day, but the years of living with AIDS have turned him into an old man.

"Hi James, my name is Dominick and I'm your nurse. How ya feeling?"

He doesn't look up at me.

"Okay, James, I'm going to help you change into your pajamas and then we'll get you some dinner. We have a great cook on staff and I think tonight its roast chicken with mashed potatoes and gravy."

He still won't talk to me, or even move. I put the clean hospital pajamas on his bed. I look at his chart and read that he's in the end-stage of AIDS, can't hold his bowels, little appetite.

I take out my stethoscope, check his heart and record it on the chart. Then I take his pulse. As I stand there, counting the beats, I look over at the bathroom. The door is open and I realize why James won't look up.

He's afraid of the mirror.

I help him into his pajamas; he keeps his head down.

"James, would you feel better if I covered the mirror?" I ask.

He nods his head "yes".

I go into the bathroom, take one of the bath towels and hang it over the mirror. I wash my hands in the sink then go back to James. I tape down his IV line and insert the IV into the port in his hand.

"Ok, James, I'm going to tell the cafeteria to send in your dinner. Would you like me to turn on the TV?"

He shakes his head 'no'.

I ask if there is anything I can do to make him comfortable. He doesn't say anything and turns on his side to face the window.

I start for the door.

"Please don't go," he says. "I could use the company."

I walk to his bed, pull up the chair and sit down. He turns over and looks directly at me. Tears roll down his cheeks. I reach out and take his hand; and as I sit by his bed waiting for him to fall asleep, I think about Jorge.

# 1994
# My New Amigo ...

It was end of my senior year at Christ Hospital School of Nursing, and I was just a few months away from graduation when I arrived at the nurses' station at 6:30 am, nervous as hell because I was about to perform a blood transfusion on a patient with AIDS anemia. My nursing instructor Miss Marcelo called me into the conference room.

"Dominick, before you meet Mr. Perez, I want you to know why I gave you this patient," she says. "It's because I know you can help him. He's having a blood transfusion because he's extreme-ly anemic, but it's not about the blood transfusion. I want you to get his story, his information. I want you to be there for him."

"I can do that."

"I'm putting you to the test," she continued.

I was eager and anxious to get started.

I headed to the transfusion room, thinking about what she said. This was scary stuff because blood transfusions are scary interventions especially for a student doing it for the first time. What I needed to do was something more than the blood transfusion.

I slowly opened the door to the transfusion room. It was brightly lit with cushioned recliner chairs lining the room. Jorge was sitting in a recliner with his eyes closed. I could see he was very sick. Although he had Kaposi Sarcoma lesions on his nose and face, he was still a very handsome man with black hair, black eyes and in great physical shape for someone in his condition.

"Hi Jorge."

He opened his eyes, looked at me and said hello.

"My name is Dominick. How you feeling, today?"

"Okay, I guess. A little weak."

"Well, we're going to take care of that right now. I'm going to give you a blood transfusion, which will give you energy in no time."

Okay? Sure."

"Let me just do a few things first. We'll have a chat and then I'm going to take your blood pressure while I do the procedure; this way I can monitor you."

This was not Jorge's first transfusion; he had done them sev-eral times before. At first, he was more help to me than I was to him. I checked his vital signs, completed all the necessary paperwork, and took the papers to the Pharmacy along with the RN from the unit. I had a supervisor verify everything and then went back to Jorge. I hung the blood on the IV pole and re-checked all the important data. I re-checked his vital signs and as instructed, I did that every 15 minutes afterwards.

While the blood is transfusing, you need to make some con-nection, engage the patient. We're taught how to do that right from nursing 101. You first start with questions like 'where were you born' and then you go to specifics by asking open-ended questions allowing people to let out their inner most feelings and concerns.

The scary part of that for a student nurse is that you never know what a patient is going to tell you. As I worked toward the specific, nearing the end of the blood transfusion, I asked him, "when you go home today, what do you feel will be your biggest concern or your biggest obstacle to overcome?"

He told me he was worried about walking his dog, a white pit bull named Ruffie who he adored more than anything in the world.

I sat there with Jorge for two hours, checked his blood pres-sure and we talked. I found out he only lived about eight blocks from me, and he loved his dog. I also found out that Jorge was gay. Jorge celebrated Ruffie's birthday every year in November. Jorge would bake him a cake, light a candle, sing Happy Birthday and blow out the candle. Then the dog would gobble the cake down.

Jorge conveyed to me that he had a problem. I was glad he felt some degree of comfort with me that he was able to open up at least a little.

"I can't walk Ruffie anymore," he told me. "He 'goes' in my house. I block off the kitchen and let him go there." Knowing how dangerous feces and dog urine was to Jorge's health and considering I lived only a few blocks away, I volunteered to help.

"I can walk Ruffie," I reassured him.

"You would do that for me?"

"Of course. I'm a dog-lover, too. We have one of our own, a wire-haired Jack Russell we call Tallulah."

"We? Are you married?"

"Well, not exactly. My partner and I live together."

"Your partner?"

"Yes."

He looked at me and realized that I was gay, too.

"What time should I come over?" I asked.

"Anytime really," Jorge said.

"Well, I have to be here at the hospital by 6:30, so how about I get to your place at 5:45."

"That would be great," Jorge said. "Thank you so much. What is your name again?"

"Dominick."

"Thank you, Dominick, thank you."

I asked Jorge for a phone number where I could best reach him in case there was a problem. I also got his address from the chart.

After a very successful transfusion, Jorge was discharged. There was a car service provided by New Jersey's AIDS organization, the Hyacinth Foundation, and Jorge took the ride home.

Ms. Marcelo was very happy when I told her Jorge would be in good hands and I would continue to work with him as best I could as long as it didn't interfere with my schoolwork.

The next morning, I went to Jorge's house. He had breakfast all ready and over flatbread sandwiches made with ham and cheese and *café con leche*- strong coffee made with steamed milk - Jorge told me about his family in Puerto Rico and his ex-lover Patrick who had left him.

He told me his lover left because he couldn't cope with Jorge's diagnosis and knowing that Jorge was eventually going to die was too much for him to bear.

I began walking Ruffie every morning.

After a couple of weeks, I learned the Student Council was running a bus trip to Atlantic City. I asked Jorge if he felt well enough to go with us. We only had 40 students and the bus held 50 people, so he decided to come along knowing he would be in the best care with 40 student nurses looking out for him.

I'm not a gambler, so we walked the boardwalk. It was the end of March and a little chilly, but we were dressed warm and took breaks whenever Jorge felt tired.

Spending that day with Jorge, I was able to understand "a day in the life" of an end-stage AIDS patient. Walking on the board-walk. Having a hot chocolate. We had a great time. The whole class embraced him, which made me feel a little better about my classmates after what happened in Psych last semester.

"How about support group meetings." I said as the bus bar-reled along the New Jersey Turnpike, "I'll go with you."

Jorge said he went a couple of times, but it wasn't his cup of tea. He wanted to spend time with me, he said.

"Can't we just hang out for coffee once in a while?"

Knowing Jorge was becoming weak, his mother, father and brother Ed took turns staying with him at his apartment in Jersey City. There were times when all of them would be there, and we would have dinner together. At first, Jorge introduced me as his nurse, but we were quickly becoming friends.

# Give Me Liberty

During the following months, Bob came with me a few times to Jorge's place and Jorge was to our home a few times, too. He especially liked Tallulah, our Jack Russell terrier. He used to call Tallulah "Lunch" because Ruffie was a Pit Bull and Tallulah looked like she could be Ruffie's lunch. We didn't dare put them together.

One night when Jorge was sick we brought him and Ruffie to our house and put Ruffie in the basement and he tore the door off the laundry room hinges. I was not angry, but I had to be cautious or poor little Tallulah would have been lunch for Ruffie that night. The next day I was able to get Jorge in to see Dr. Mangia. I really liked Dr. Mangia right away and thought, maybe some day I would like to work for him. But God was leading me in a different direction; I just didn't know that yet.

Taking care of Jorge and trying to bring up my failing grades at the same time was more than a full-time job, but those times were rewarding in so many ways. The main part of this learning experience was that it taught me how to multi-task, something every nurse has to do every day of his or her life. Being there for Jorge actually helped pull me through this rough time at school, because it was a reminder of how much people living with AIDS were going to need me.

Jorge also inspired me to strive harder and reach my goal. When someone is very ill, and they look you in the eye and say, "I can't do this without your help," you just have to step up. This is why I credit God and Ms. Marcelo for bringing Jorge into my life. Jorge is one of the main reasons I knew I had to do whatever it takes to get through this senior year of nursing school and be successful in my new career as an AIDS Nurse.

On Tuesday May 10, I woke up extra early to take the final exam. This was the final, final exam. After failing test one with a 56 in early February, I busted my butt the next three tests to bring my average up. I was able to pass all three tests after that first one, however my average was still under 70 percent.

I met Jorge in March of this year, and was feeling pretty good because the day before meeting him I had taken test two and scored a 78. But when you add 56 and 78 and divide by two you get an average of 67 percent. I had to work really hard because I did not want to go into the final exam of my senior year with a failing average.

On test three I got a 70 percent and test four a whopping 72 percent. I thought I was going to die. After three full years I just could not fail out now. I needed a 76 on the final exam in order to get my diploma. I went to bed early the night before the final to ensure that I would be well rested.

The next morning, I left the house at 7 am even though the exam was at 8:30. I dropped Bob off at the Pavonia Avenue PATH station. He kissed me and wished me luck. I was shaking like a leaf all the way to school.

I parked my car and walked over to the Christ Hospital Chapel. They have a podium there with a book on it where you can write a special intention and have people pray for you. I went into the chapel and wrote in the book, "Dear God, I have to take my final exam today and I need a 76 to pass the nursing course so I can be a Nurse. I am not asking for an 80, or a 75, I need a 76 and that is it," signed Dominick P. Varsalone.

I dropped down to my knees feeling a bit uncomfortable asking for God's help again and I prayed and prayed until it was time to go to class. I walked out of the hospital chapel and ran into Jean, whom I became friends with during my freshman year.

She had been a volunteer at the hospital for more years than any other volunteer and when she learned of my decision to work as an AIDS Nurse, she was a tremendous support to me. I asked her if she would say a special prayer for me that day, too, as I was going into the final exam in very poor shape.

I walked through the underground tunnel between the hospital and the school of nursing telling myself, just pass this exam and you will never have to do this again. I went through the tunnel to try to avoid running into any of my classmates because I was too nervous to hear about how nervous they were. I think there was only one or two students going into the final with a failing average.

As I sat in the brightly-lit room shaking with my #2 lead pencils in hand, I remember not looking at anyone or talking to anyone. I was too nervous to even talk to my study group pals. When all 37 students were seated, Mrs. Growney said in a soft voice "Okay class, you can begin, good luck to all of you."

I took a deep breath, said a silent prayer and two hours later it was pencils down. I swear I have never seen two hours go by so quickly in my life. I turned in my paper and ran out to the front steps of the school hyperventilating. The smokers in the group were already lit up. Doreen and a few other people were crying thinking they had failed the final. I was nervous because I found the questions on this exam to be really easy and I remembered that was how I felt after test one when I got a 56. This sent me into a panic. We all hung out on the steps for about an hour and went back inside only to be told by the administrators that they had to recalculate the final exam results and we would not get the grades until Friday.

I went home in a panic almost wanting a cigarette after having quit eight years ago. When Bob came home he was expecting there would be something for dinner, but I just could not bring myself to cook. He went to the fridge and scrounged up some leftovers while I sat at the dining room table sobbing. He kept saying, "How do you know you failed?"

Of course I could not answer that question. I had no idea how I did but I did know I was not feeling at all good about it.

Three agonizing days passed and when I woke up on Friday, I felt dazed. Bob was very reassuring as he always is. He gave me a kiss and said Happy Birthday and don't worry you passed. I just know they won't fail you on your birthday.

I walked over to Jorge's apartment that morning instead of driving because I needed to clear my head and I was not under any time constraints. When I got there Jorge had one of those ham and cheese flat sandwiches ready for me. I walked Ruffie and ate my flat ham and cheese sandwich. Jorge looked right at me and said, "for all you have done for me, you will be rewarded."

"I just want a 76 on the exam, that's all," I said.

Jorge walked me to the door and said, "Good luck Papi and Happy Birthday."

I took a slow walk back home. I went into the house and my phone was ringing. I decided to pick it up and I'm glad I did. "Dominick. It's Doreen," her excited voice said. "I passed, I passed! I can't believe it. I am a Nurse."

I asked her about the others and she said, "Winston and Maria are already here and they passed too."

Great. I was happy for all of them, but I kept thinking I was probably the only one who didn't make it. By this time, I was really anxious. On the way to the school I was thinking about Frankie and Cal, Matt, Pasquale, Ben, Rich, and so many others I also thought of my cousin Marge. They would all be proud of me. I most especially was thinking about Bob and the three years of torture I had put him through.

If I fail this exam, I would not be able to look at him and tell him. I parked the car, ran into the school, got to the bulletin board, found my Social Security number, and next to that, written in the last column: "76".

I must have read it a dozen times.

I was emotionless.

I did not go out the front door to tell everyone I passed. I went downstairs and walked through the underground tunnel to the hospital directly to the chapel and wrote in the spiral-bound notebook "Thank you God. Thanks for the 76."

I left the chapel and saw Jean. I gave her a kiss on the cheek and a big hug. "I did it!" I told her. Jean smiled and said, "I know you did because God answers all of my prayers."

I ran across Palisade Avenue back toward the school, right to Doreen, Winston and Maria who would not go home until they found out if I passed. We did the biggest group hug and everyone was laughing and crying all at the same time. These were tears of happiness as our hard work had paid off. All 37 students who made it to the final exam passed and although that should signify the end of school it was not over yet. There was National League of Nursing (NLN) exams, the exit exam, and sessions with our NLN mentor.

I had to go back into the school to see who my mentor was. As I walked up to that bulletin board I checked one last time to be sure that 76 was next to my name and not someone else's. Then I looked up at the mentorship sheet and saw that ROC would be my faculty mentor for preparation for the state board exam. I would have to deal with that on Monday because I was going home to celebrate what would be one of the best birthdays of my life. I made a bunch of phone calls the first one to Bob who said "Congratulations Honey! Don't cook anything; I am taking you out tonight for your birthday, and we can celebrate your becoming a nurse."

On Monday all the students went back to school where we were met with a coffee and bagel reception. We all had to sit with our faculty mentors and devise a plan of study for the exit exam and the State Board exam. My mentor was Rose O'Connor. I really liked her. For the three years at school she was my clinical instructor for one rotation and a specialist in Orthopedics.

I was especially fond of that rotation because I applied my ability to repair freight trains all those years to the traction devices, which were a piece of cake to figure out. Some of the other students had a difficult time with Mrs. O because she was a tough sell and she did not buy any bull from anyone, not even me, and I am the master of "If you can't dazzle them with your brilliance baffle them with your bullshit."

Many of the other students thought Mrs. O or "ROC" as she was affectionately known, was too rigid. ROC was tough, but a great teacher.

It was my turn to go to the dungeon; her small office was in the school basement across from the skills lab. Dark paneling was the design. It was hot and stuffy and room for only her chair and desk and the chair I was sitting on. Our conversation went something like this:

ROC: "So you barely passed I see?"
Me: "Yeah barely 70.1, which is .1 more than I prayed for."
ROC: "You do realize that you have to come up with a plan that will convince me, and the Director of Nursing that you will pass the State Board exam?" she said. "I want you to explain to me in detail what your plan of action

will be and if I don't think it is good enough believe you me, mister, I will crack that whip."

Me: "Well, thank you, Mrs. O'Connor, all my life others have had more confidence in me than I had in myself until now. Here is my plan."

I had mapped out in detail everything I set out to do to get this job done. I spent the entire weekend planning my study time and reviewing every book, notebook and slip of paper I wrote anything on for three years and organized it into a study plan. ROC was so surprised she said to me.

"Well I have to tell you Dominick (she never calls students by their first name). This is the first time in all of my years here at the school of nursing that the student came up with a tougher plan of study than I had planned for them. I think you will be just fine, provided that you stick to this plan."

I left there sweating and not from the heat.

From mid-May until Graduation Day, I studied every day. I started out by re-writing all of my notes into a study notebook; every note from the last three years was re-written because they say if you write it, read it and review it you will be more likely to remember it.

I then made flash cards and carried them with me wherever I went. If I was in the supermarket on a long line I would whip out the cards and study. I think I did more studying in the post office than just about anywhere else. Most of my time I spent in my car at Liberty State Park. I would take all of my notes, books and some relaxation tapes and head over there. When I was tired I would walk around the park to clear my head of negative thoughts and take in some fresh air. (As fresh as it gets in New Jersey.)

The most beautiful site to see when you are walking by the Hudson River is the New York City Skyline. When I was in high school, from 1971 to 1974, the World Trade Center's Twin Towers were being built, and I kept saying to myself if people can build those huge buildings then I can be a nurse. The Statue of Liberty, which you can see from Liberty State Park in Jersey City, just a short ride from Bob's and my house, reminded me that people came to this country aspiring for a better life. I was born in this country; and I, too, wanted a better life.

I felt it all coming together and even the most mundane tasks and the toughest obstacles I faced in nursing school were beginning to make sense. I felt as if a light bulb had gone off in my head and I began to question how I could not see it when I was in school studying. I now know it is because I had to take everything I learned and become my own person.

I had to develop myself as Dominick Varsalone, AIDS Nurse, and that meant the same compassionate care I give to my friends and family members, I will give to my patients.

# 103 Women and Me

It was a beautiful June day, sunny, not too hot, and what could be better than graduating from nursing school?

Bob and I went to pick up my sister Alice from the airport. Mom, Dad, my brother and his wife were also coming to the graduation along with Bob's mom and dad who came in from Iowa a few days ago. Jorge was there along with Teresa. There were lots of pictures taken outside before the ceremony.

I remember running up to Barbara Davey and Brenda Pelicano to give them a big hug and a great big thank you for giving me the nursing school application that day. Barbara was looking at me so proud and asked if I wanted to meet Bishop John Shelby Spong, the Episcopal Bishop of Newark. It was exciting to meet a Bishop; and the closest I will ever get to royalty.

Graduation was held at the Old Bergen Church in Jersey City. Everyone who had anything to do with the school was there including House Mother Cathe Killman, Librarian Kate Vargo, and all the instructors. They lined us up in alphabetical order and we walked down the aisle accompanied by *The Graduation March*. The Bishop and clergy led the way, followed by dignitaries, award presenters, the instructors and 37 graduates; 12 men with red roses in our lapels, and 25 women with red long-stem roses in their hands. Our faculty advisor Mrs. Growney led us in.

We got to our seats and on each seat was a program and candle, which was to be lit for the Nurse's Pledge. I don't remember who our speakers were because I was so nervous thinking the diploma would not be in the folder when I got it and all of this was just a dream. I was doing well up until they played *Wind Beneath my Wings* and I totally lost it. Doreen, who was sitting next to me, slapped me on the shoulder and said, "get a grip, girlfriend." She could always make me laugh. The Wind Beneath my Wings was the song that was playing on the day my railroad mentor, Walter "Red" Kimball died. He would have been so proud that I made it to this day.

After a few more speeches, graduation pins and diplomas were handed out to the graduates. I wanted to wear my AIDS ribbon pin but they would not allow it because it was not considered part of the uniform. I pleaded with Mrs. Fasano that I had promised my friend Jorge I would wear it for him."

"Dominick if you wear that pin, I will yank you right out of the line and hold your diploma," she said.

I thought after three years of nursing school, "Hell, I should be able to wear a diamond tiara." But I complied, at least until after I received my pin and diploma. As I walked back to my seat, I pulled that red ribbon out of my pocket and stuck it right under my red rose. Let them try to take this diploma away from me now, they wouldn't be able to pry it out of my cold dead hands.

I got back to my seat and showed Doreen my red ribbon pin and she said, "You go girl." It was time for the awards that go to all the students with the highest grades. I wasn't paying much attention because I was too busy being "Mr. Defiant" with my red ribbon.

The awards were announced: The Gloria Larsen Lobin Award, Nursing Achievement Award, NLN Leadership award, Student Council Award, and the Bishop of Newark Award. Barbara Davey got up and introduced the Bishop who said, "I am here to present the Christ Hospital School of Nursing Bishop of Newark Award for May 1994. Let it be known by all who read this that the Bishop of Newark Award is presented to the graduate who consistently demonstrates empathy, understanding and concern for all his patients and is a very caring person. This year's award is presented to: Dominick Varsalone."

There were screams and shouts and loud applause and I was totally oblivious that the Bishop had just announced my name. Doreen was squeezing my arm, saying "get up there, get up there, it's you, you won it."

The moment I realized I won that award the first thing I thought was oh my God, I have this red ribbon on now and Mrs. Fasano is going to take the award away from me, but it was too late to do anything. As I made my way up to the stage, the Bishop was telling everyone that this was the first year in the school's 104-year history that the award went to a male student.

When he presented me with the award he shook my hand and told me that he was very happy to see the red ribbon on my uniform and that it was a sign of my deep compassion for the work I was about to embark upon. When I got back to my seat, it was time to light the candle and say my pledge.

*"I solemnly pledge myself before God and in the presence of this assembly to pass my life in purity and to practice my profession faithfully. I shall abstain from whatever is deleterious and mischievous, and I shall do all in my power to maintain and elevate the standard of my profession and will hold in confidence all personal matters committed to my keeping and all my family affairs coming to my knowledge in the practice of my calling. I shall be loyal to my work and devoted toward the welfare of those committed to my care."*

We sang *God Bless America* and walked out of the church. Family and friends joined the graduates downstairs for punch and cookies. We had pictures taken for the newspaper; my picture with the Bishop was in the *Jersey Journal,* too.

When the congratulatory photos, handshakes and kisses were done, all the graduates went their separate ways to celebrate and party. People kept telling me how proud they were, but none more proud than Bob. The best part of the whole day was being able to fall asleep in the arms of the most amazing man in the world. If it had not been for Bob's continued support and encouragement, I probably would have quit nursing school. When I woke up on June 11· all I could think about was Mrs. O'Connor's final words to me:

*"You do realize that you have to come up with a plan that will convince me and the Director of Nursing that you will pass the State Board exam."*

I knew I had to get right back to studying. I did allow myself a break because family was in town through the weekend. I was having my party at the church on Sunday, Alice was going home Sunday night, and Bob's parents were leaving on Tuesday. At Grace Church on Sunday, there were over 120 people in church for the service and several more came afterwards. It was the biggest crowd at Grace Lutheran in years.

Bob and I drove his parents to the airport Tuesday morning and I immediately went to work studying for the State Board exam. I wanted to take it as soon as possible after the study time was over so that I wouldn't forget what I learned. I called the Board of Nursing to set the date and chose July 18. My friend Alice Gruenberg from Temple B'Nai Jacob in Jersey City told me that the number 18 in the Jewish faith is a lucky number.

# ROC Around the Clock

For the next month, I studied 12 hours a day with the vision of Mrs. Rose O'Connor standing behind me cracking a whip. I was doing great with my studying and every morning, afternoon and evening, I'd check up on Jorge and walk Ruffie. I did take a little bit of a break on July 4, with a little party in the backyard. By the end of the evening, I noticed Jorge was looking really pale.

I noticed his breathing was slightly labored and I asked him if he wanted to stay at our house with us that night. We pulled out the couch bed in the living room and for the next couple of days Jorge stayed with us.

I went to walk the dog every day and I studied at home for those days. On July 8 we went to see Dr. Mangia, who asked me to take Jorge to St. Francis hospital as a direct admit. Jorge had to have a blood transfusion and some really serious tests done.

I was torn as to how much time I should spend with Jorge at the hospital and how much time I needed to spend on my studies. Jorge knew I was not able to stay all day with him, so he called Jeff, Louie, Nelson, Enrique and a few other friends and asked if they could visit him. Jorge's friends were very committed to him. Everyone who knew Jorge loved him and that is why it was so easy for us to become friends. As a professional, maybe I should have created some distance the patient. But Jorge was special and Bob and I adored him.

Just about a week before my test on July 18, the unthinkable happened. Jorge had to remain at St Francis hospital with severe anemia, and his lesions had spread to the lymph nodes in his groin area. When I got to the hospital I assured Jorge that if he stayed strong he could get through this rough time like he always had done in the past. I also decided that I needed to take a ride to the Christ Hospital chapel and put Jorge's name in that spiral book. While I was there I put another request in the book asking for a passing grade on the State Boards.

I went through the tunnel under Palisade Avenue and went to see my advisor "The ROC" and anyone else who might be in the school that day, to tell them I was ready for the State Board exam. ROC gave me the biggest hug, and told me she would also be praying for Jorge. She knew this meant a great deal to me.

I spent much of the weekend relaxing and not studying. I also visited Jorge frequently since St. Francis Hospital was right down the street from me. Jorge's parents and his brother Ed came in while he was in the hospital so I knew he was in good hands. They stayed at Jorge's apartment but we also gave them a key to our home because it was a short walk from the hospital for Pito and Elsa.

# The Impossible Dream

When July 18 came I was ready to greet my challenge. I got up early and paced around the house nervously. I showered and got dressed, ate breakfast and saw Bob off to work. My emotions were running wild.

When I arrived at the testing site in Newark it hit me that we would be taking this exam on the computer. The class of 1994 was the first class to do this. I began to panic. I sat down at my assigned desk in the testing room along with nine other graduate nurses. I said a short prayer and began answering the questions. After almost two hours I looked up and I was the only one still testing. I had no way of knowing how long it would be before I was done. Suddenly the computer shut down and the words "You have completed the exam" appeared on the screen.

I left the campus, walked to the train, got to Jersey City and went directly to Christ Hospital Chapel. I wrote another note in that spiral binder, which was now filled mostly with notes to God from me.

The next morning, Bob and I were driving to Canada for a week. I had to have a vacation once the exam was completed and I was hoping to get my test results shortly after my return.

Before we left, we stopped at the hospital to see Jorge. I know Dr. Mangia wanted to do a biopsy of the lymph nodes lesions, but I did not want him to do that. It had been my experience that once they invade the area the cancer spreads faster. I also knew that they could not actually give a diagnosis of KS unless a biopsy was done to confirm it was actually KS and not something else. Needless to say we all knew it was KS; nevertheless; it had to be done. I told Jorge that he could refuse the test, but he chose to have the biopsy.

Quebec was beautiful and relaxing, just what the doctor ordered for this nurse-to-be. The weather was beautiful, cool and dry. I am so glad that I took French in high school. My teacher Edward T. McGhee thought I would make a great Translator for the United Nations. Of course that dream was not fulfilled. I guess it was a schoolboy fantasy. Bob was really impressed with my communication in French while we were in Canada, and I had fun trying to get us here and there.

When we returned that following Sunday, there was a stack of mail on the counter. Our friend Robert Mason was taking care of our cats, Bette and Joan, (named for those movie actress divas Bette Davis and Joan Crawford) and our Jack Russell terrier Tallulah (Bankhead) while we were gone. We walked into the house, dropped the bags, took a quick peek through the mail, and there it was, a large yellow envelope from the State Board of Nursing with my test results. I started to shake and told Bob to open it for me.

Bob said "You have to open it; I can't do that for you." As usual Bob was right. I had to own the result. Still I was trembling. I carefully ripped open the envelope at the top and slid out the letter. I took a very deep breath and then opened my eyes to read what it said. All I needed to see was the first word, Congratulations! And I started to cry like a baby.

Bob of course had no idea if I was crying because I passed or failed and he kept saying, "What did it say? What did it say?" Then he grabbed the paper out of my hand and read it out loud, "Congratulations you have passed the Nursing State Board Exam. You may now work as a Registered Nurse." Then he gave me a big hug saying, "Congratulations honey, I knew you could do it!"

I called Robert Mason to thank him for watching our pets and told him the news; he was elated. I called my family, my study-group pals, Virginia, the Ladies of Grace, and my friends. Bob and I unpacked our suitcases, threw a load of clothes in the washing machine, and practically ran to see Jorge in Saint Francis Hospital.

When I told him the good news he lit up like a Christmas tree. "Congratulations Papi," he said, "you deserve it."

Now as a registered nurse with a license, I asked Jorge how he was doing, and what the doctor said. He told me that they did the biopsy and confirmed that it was Kaposi's Sarcoma (the AIDS Cancer).

Jorge had spent almost two weeks in St. Francis Hospital and he was ready to come home. His parents and his brother came up to take care of his apartment and to see that Ruffie was walked and fed while Bob and I were on vacation. They invited me for dinner the last night before going back to Puerto Rico. Jorge's dad, Pito was a really great cook; he made pastilles and empanadas, along with other tasty treats that caused me to overeat.

The next morning, I drove them all to the airport and they hugged and thanked me for taking care of Jorge. His mom Elsa cried and his dad Pito told me that anytime Bob and I wanted to go to Puerto Rico for a vacation we had a place to stay at their beach house.

# Ruffie goes to Oz

Because of the blood transfusion, Jorge was feeling a little bit better. However, it was getting harder and harder for Jorge to care for Ruffie. It was time for me to start talking to Jorge about how we could find a home for his dog, a very difficult conversation.

The gay community had a program in New York called Pets of People with AIDS, (we didn't have one in New Jersey yet) where volunteer pet sitters care for the pets of people with AIDS while they are in the hospital.

I reached out to my friends and asked if anyone could take care of Ruffie. My friend Angel and his partner Luis who lived in downtown Jersey City volunteered to care for Ruffie and told Jorge he could visit any time. It was heartbreaking to see Jorge say goodbye to Ruffie. Imagine Dorothy coming back from Oz without Toto. Still, Jorge had to do something and having people that we know who lived close by volunteer to care for Ruffie was a stroke of good luck. Of course there were visitation rights, anytime Jorge wanted to.

# Pounding the Pavement

The next two months my main mission was to find a job now that I had the certificate that said I could work as a nurse. I had to purchase malpractice insurance first. Imagine paying money for insurance before you earn any back. I asked Dawn, and others who graduated before me if there were openings, especially in AIDS Care. Unfortunately, there was a serious lack of jobs in nursing.

I called South Amboy wondering if I could work with Marylou and Peggy like I did the summer between my first and second year of school. I picked up the newspapers every day and searched all over until one day at the end of September I found out from Keith, one of the guys I graduated with, that they were looking for a Psych Nurse at JCMC, the Jersey City Medical Center.

I jumped at the opportunity to work because Bob had been footing the bill way too long. I drove to the Medical Center on Montgomery Street not far from where I grew up, and went directly to the Director of Nursing. She was impressed with my Psych score on the NLN exam, which was in the 97 percentile. I left JCMC feeling pretty good and wondering how long it would take to get called back.

It turns out I did not have to wait long. Two days later I got the call to come and start work. The orientation would be the following Monday. Bob and I went out that night to celebrate with our friend Lou Squitieri and his friend, Nelson. That night Lou, Nelson, Bob and I spoke mostly about me. They felt that this new job might not be right because I wanted to specialize in AIDS Care. But two months had gone by since I passed the Board Exam and this was the only job available.

So, I took the job. I started the hospital's orientation and according to the schedule; I would be working on the Psych Unit after 3 months of Psych Orientation. I was getting paid a full salary to watch and learn.

Yes, there would be more tests: Pharmacology tests, and basic skills tests like tying a "Posey Jacket" to restrain a violent patient. I had piles of paperwork to fill out and the whole process was like being in school again. It was only Wednesday and I was already exhausted.

When I got home the phone rang. It was Stephen, and his partner Richard are our dear friends from the Garden State Gay Bowling Organization (GSGBO). He said, "I'm calling to ask you if you got a job, yet?"

"Just this past Monday I started a job on the Psych unit at JCMC," I told him.

"Too bad," Stephen said. "My client, Michael Delsordo is opening a new AIDS facility in Newark called Broadway House. He is looking for nurses who want to work in AIDS Care."

This job sounded perfect. At the end of our conversation, I told Stephen I was definitely interested even though I had just started my first job as a nurse already. I asked him if he could get me an interview with Mr. Delsordo and he said, "yes".

I was nearly out of breath explaining to Bob my chat with Stephen. I was uncertain what I should do, and I had a huge decision to make if this new opportunity came to fruition.

Bob and I were just about ready to settle in for the night. Tallulah was sitting on my lap looking at me with her head tilted as if she knew it was Stephen we were talking about.

The phone rang. It was Stephen telling me that Mr. Delsordo wanted to know if I could come Thursday to interview for the job. I looked at Bob and he nodded "yes!" so I got the address and was there at 4:30 on Thursday.

I worked all day Thursday at the JCMC, but my mind was on Broadway House. I was wondering once again what door was about to open for me, and in what direction my life would be headed next.

I had to go to North Newark on Bloomfield Ave. to a small office above a candy store. I thought for sure I was in the wrong place. I paced around outside, looking for a sign or even a cardboard note that said Broadway House, but there was nothing. I really did not know what else to do so I rang the only bell with no name on it and was buzzed in. I walked slowly up one flight of steps and was met at the door by a woman. My first thought was, "She doesn't look like her name is Michael Delsordo. I had to ask anyway," "Hi, my name is Dominick Varsalone and I'm looking for Michael Delsordo?"

"Well you are in the right place so come on in," she said. "My name is Tawana and I am Mr. Delsordo's administrative assistant. Have a seat and someone will be right with you."

I looked around feeling a bit nervous. There was a small reception area with lots of bookshelves and a desk for Tawana.

There were also two offices with both doors closed and next to that, a very small bathroom. The reception area was brightly lit with a row of windows facing Bloomfield Avenue.

I liked her right away and felt comfortable enough to ask my stupid question, "Excuse me Tawana, I know you are very busy, but is this Broadway House?"

Tawana laughed and said, "This is the temporary office space for Broadway House," I felt foolish but Tawana continued, "Ms. O'Neil will see you as soon as she is off the phone, and the two Mikes will interview you as soon as they get back."

Carol O'Neil invited me into her small office and told me she was the Assistant Director of Nursing, and would not be doing the hiring. She told me to relax, and I did. We had a very nice conversation. Carol set the stage very well for me and told me I was exactly the type of nurse they wanted. Their requirements were a new Nursing School grad who, in their personal lives experienced a friend or family member with AIDS, and who has a passion to do something about it. Carol then asked me to tell her something about me, and how I thought I would fit that description.

I gave her the abbreviated version of my life with Bob, life as a railroad worker, and how I felt I was spiritually guided into nursing, especially into AIDS Care. She smiled and asked if I had any questions about the job. Yes, I said. I wanted to know if there were any testing requirements like what I had been experiencing at JCMC the last four days.

Carol laughed and said, "Honey if you got this far you will do just fine. We are going to teach you everything you need to know." Her words made it sound like I was already hired. Then again, when I told her about my orientation having already started at JCMC she said, "If you like our offer and accept this job, all you need to do is go there tomorrow and tell them you decided to take a different offer. It happens every year with nurses right out of nursing school, especially with those who are looking to specialize."

I knew she was right because I remembered Ms. Marcelo telling me that I may have to work in Medical/Surgical Nursing for a year before I got to specialize, and here I had two offers in specialties. When Mike Delsordo and the other Mike came back to the office, Carol jumped up and said, "You have this poor guy sitting here with me for almost an hour! I already took care of the interview for you, and I decided we would hire him."

I was shocked at what she had said, and the four of us went into the other office, which was larger and had only one desk. The other Mike extended his hand and said, "Hi I'm Michael Nelson, Director of Nursing." Mr. Delsordo looked at me over his glasses and said, "You don't need to convince me of anything. I'm only the Executive Director around here and I just do what Mike and Carol tell me to do when it comes to nursing. Besides, Stephen and I had a nice long conversation about you last night and he's my lawyer so I guess I better approve."

I must have had my jaw wide open at this sudden shower of approvals. Carol looked at Mike Delsordo and said, "Mike and I will take Dominick to the "Big House," and talk to him on the way about our offer." Mike nodded "yes".

We got into his car, I sat in the back and they took me to Broadway House, where I was about to start my career as an AIDS Nurse.

We arrived a few minutes later to the back of a huge white building. It almost looked like a City Hall Building. I found out later that it was originally the home of Mutual Benefit Life Insurance Company, then when they moved to a larger building in the downtown area of Newark the building was turned into a high school for boys. As we entered the hallway, there was a magnificent ceiling and marble floors and walls that seemed to go on forever.

Everything else in the building was still under reconstruction. On the north side of the building they were building another level with a walking bridge to get from one side to the next. Michael Nelson asked me, "So what do you think?" I was so amazed and yet still a little confused, I just couldn't find any words to say at that moment.

He then told me, "This is going to be the place in all of New Jersey for people living with AIDS to come for their care, and you, my friend, can be the first Nurse we hire to care for them." We toured a little more and I was told where everything was going to be, and that Broadway House would be a long-term care facility exclusively for people with AIDS where they could either recover from acute illness and go home to their families or come to die in peace, and with dignity. Now it was back to the office where I signed the papers.

At home, Bob and I talked about the pay difference between Broadway House and JCMC. JCMC paid a much higher salary than Broadway House, but Bob and I agreed, a person has to love what they do, even if it's for less money. Bob assured me we would be fine financially.

The next day, I went to the Director of Nursing at JCMC and told her I had a different offer that I really wanted to take because I would be working with AIDS patients. She was not at all angry like I thought she would be. She told me, "Follow your heart and your dream, that is always first and foremost." She gave me a hug and wished me luck.

I began training for my work at Broadway House. I first worked with Tawana by helping her put together the Policy and Procedure Manuals. Meanwhile, Mike and Carol were busy hiring the rest of the staff. By Thanksgiving, we were training with one of the most wonderful nurses I have ever met, Nancy Scangarello at Saint Michael's Medical Center's Peter Ho Clinic in Newark.

It was during this time that my good friend Rich died of AIDS. He was 42. His sister Elsie called me with the news. It seems that ever since his beloved Ben died a year ago in May, Rich never recovered from his loss. It would seem he gave up the fight, but that's not the case. Rich and I had many conversations after Ben died, and Rich told me even though he had HIV, he wanted to keep fighting.

Rich's sisters loved him very much. They were his caretakers and did their best to keep his friends informed of his health. God Bless you, my friend, you were special to me.

# Hello Broadway House

I was writing procedures for Broadway House and taking classes at St. Michael's Medical Center on treatments for AIDS patients. Nurse Nancy, an AIDS Nurse at the Peter Ho clinic in Newark, an outpatient clinic for people with HIV, was my instructor. She worked with Dr. George Perez, who was in charge.

When we met, I asked Dr. Perez if he spelled his first name with a "J" or a "G" and he asked me why? I told him I have a friend named Jorge Perez who is living in my home. Dr. Perez and I developed an immediate connection.

Dr. Perez and Nurse Nancy taught all the nurses hired for Broadway House. We were blessed to be taught by the best.

The learning process continued at my new job where every-day was something new, different and exciting. I was eager to soak up every bit of information I could, so I would be prepared for the patients' arrivals when the new facility was approved by the State.

Meanwhile, Jorge could no longer afford the rent for his apartment, so even though he didn't want to go back to Puerto Rico, he felt he had no choice. I helped him pack and ship most of his belongings.

Together, we shipped the larger items to his family and left his clothes and a few personal belongings. Jorge and I talked a lot about his health and what he would do in Puerto Rico, because the specialized care he needed was not readily available where he would be.

It was then that I thought maybe Bob and I could invite Jorge to live with us. When Bob came home from work I asked if we could take Jorge in, so that I could care for him and he would be close to St. Francis Hospital. Jorge had already spent several nights at our home during recovery periods after his stays at St. Francis, and he was never a burden, so Bob gave his approval.

I asked Jorge the next day if he would like to stay with us and he was so happy he hugged me and wept. That entire week we packed Jorge's furniture and shipped it to Puerto Rico. We packed his clothes and Jorge moved in.

On the bad days I was right there with him as his support system and on the good days Jorge was out being Jorge, meeting new people with his beautiful smile, sense of humor and striking good looks. When he was feeling really good, Jorge would even have dinner ready for Bob and me when we got home from work. Traditional Puerto Rican dishes that his dad cooked plus rice and beans made in Jorge's rice pot, and pineapple upside-down cake or flan for dessert. Jorge was an amazing cook.

For Thanksgiving, Bob and I went to Iowa to visit his family and Jorge stayed at the house and took care of the pets. Tallulah especially was great for Jorge, she was small, unlike Ruffie, and Jorge had a great affection for animals. He loved and took care of Tallulah the same way he took care of Ruffie. When we returned, Jorge helped Bob and I decorate the house for Christmas and the annual party that would follow at the beginning of January. What I didn't know was, that while we were in Iowa, Jorge went out shopping to buy us a Christmas present.

Christmas morning, we were all in front of the tree opening presents. Bob and I were not expecting Jorge to get us anything, but he did, a white ceramic canister set for the kitchen.

By the end of the evening, I noticed Jorge was having some difficulty breathing, so we called Dr. Mangia's office the next day, and set up a breathing treatment to be done at St. Michael's where I was training.

Nurse Nancy allowed me to stay with Jorge while he was getting his treatment. Everyone at Broadway House and the Peter Ho Clinic was understanding of what I was going through with Jorge. They allowed me to take him home and have the rest of the day off with him.

We had our annual party on December 30. We did not want to do it on New Year's Eve or New Year's Day because many people already have their own plans. We asked Jorge to invite some of his friends to the party, which is how we met Nelson and Enrique. We already met Jeff and Luis and a few others along with about 40 of our friends.

It was a nice party, mostly quiet conversation and holiday music playing in the background. Most of my time was spent serving the guests, watching out for Jorge who was looking a little weaker every day, and telling everyone about my new job at Broadway House. The State Inspectors were going to be there on January 3 to give final approval for opening.

# 1995
# Bad Boy, Wha'cha Gonna Do?

Jorge had mentioned to me that he never had a surprise birthday party, so right after the new year, Bob and I sprang into action planning Jorge's surprise birthday party for January 13.

The State Inspectors came January 3, as planned; and we were all excited to get started on our respective jobs. Unfortunately, the State failed us, and our opening would be delayed.

On Friday, January 13, Jeff and Luis took Jorge out for the day, so we could decorate and prepare. It worked out really well and when they arrived back at our place, we all surprised Jorge. When he came in, he said, "oh no!" Many of his friends were there with cards and gifts, hugs, and kisses. There were balloons, party hats, lots of food and a birthday cake.

Jorge had an old car; it was parked outside our house without license plates. We were always worried that it would be spotted and get towed away. The party was just getting started and Jorge was feeling a little weak and sitting on the couch when the door-bell rang.

I went to the door and a handsome police officer stood there.

"Who owns that car outside without license plates?" the cop asked in a gruff and angry voice.

Jorge looked scared out of his mind.

The cop walked right up to Jorge and as the music was start-ed, began to undress. The party was hot but not nearly as hot as our cop/stripper. What a body and what a performance. He pulled off the prank – and his clothes, perfectly.

Jorge was a very happy man that day.

Jorge stayed in bed all day Saturday and developed intracta-ble hiccups. I felt bad, even a little guilty, because it seemed like the party wiped him out. The thing about intractable hiccups is that you cannot stop them. At first Jorge was laughing every time he would try to say something and then he would hiccup and laugh. After a few hours of this I began to worry, I remembered a technique I learned in nursing school called cupping. So I helped Jorge roll over on his stomach and began to gently tap on his back with cupped hands I did this for hours cupping and rubbing his back. I sat on the bed next to Jorge taking breaks in between cupping and massaging his back and the hiccups stopped, and Jorge fell asleep.

Bob came up from downstairs and asked if I was ready for bed and I told him I was going to sleep next to Jorge in case he woke up and the hiccups started again.

On Sunday morning Bob and I went to church and Jorge rested all day feeling pretty weak. He had developed a cough, too.

Opening day for Broadway House was set for Monday January 16, and while there were no patients in the beds, we went through the motions as if there were. We ran fire drills, performed mock codes, and practiced filling out paperwork for initial assessments just as if there were people in the beds.

The following weekend Jorge had made plans to go to Puerto Rico to be the godfather for his nephew, Christopher's christening.

Dr. Mangia was back from vacation and finally had a chance to look at Jorge's blood work taken the day after Christmas. He called Jorge telling him he had double PCP Pneumonia, the AIDS pneumonia. He recommended that Jorge not go to Puerto Rico, but Jorge was not having it.

Dr. Mangia said to me, "Dominick I can't stop him from going, but you and I both know he may not return. You need to prepare for this scenario."

I trusted Dr. Mangia and knew he was right. I spoke again to Jorge, to no avail. This was something he had to do, he said.

Jorge was leaving Thursday evening to go to the airport. Jeff and Luis were always there for Jorge and they came for the ride with us. We saw Jorge to the gate, waved goodbye, all the while thinking we may never see him again.

Jeff and Luis were very quiet on the way home, they came in for coffee and cake that Bob had made the night before to see if we could get Jorge to eat something. We all agreed to do our best to stay in touch if Jorge did not return from Puerto Rico. It was a solemn evening with many tears and many hugs of thanks to Jorge for bringing us together.

The christening was that Saturday, and on Sunday I got a call from Jorge's brother, Ed, that they had taken Jorge to a hospital in Puerto Rico. Ed told me they did not even know what medications to give him and they did not have the routine IV Bactrim, they only had it in pill form, and Jorge was having difficulty swallowing. I knew I had to go down there and take care of Jorge. The nurses there did not know what to do about dressing the sores he had developed on his upper legs from the KS. Jorge also developed lymphedema and lymph fluid was building up in his body causing his ankles and lower legs to swell.

I went to work on Monday and there were still no patients admitted, so I asked Mr. Nelson and Ms. O'Neil if I could take some time off without pay on Thursday and Friday to go to Puerto Rico and help Jorge. They approved with an okay from Mr. Delsordo. I knew I had made the right decision when I took the job. Truly, they were people who cared about people with AIDS.

When I got to Puerto Rico, Ed picked me up at the airport and we went directly to the hospital where I taught the nurses how to dress Jorge's wounds. While I was with Jorge those three days we talked a lot. For whatever reason, he wanted to go back to New Jersey to die; he did not want to die in Puerto Rico. I told

Jorge I did not think that was possible. I am not sure if he was just uncomfortable with the lack of care he was getting there or if he just did not want his family to see him die this way. I told him I would talk with his brother Ed.

Ed was in the military and high up in the ranking. He was also a Navy Medic. Ed told me he would work on it and see what he could do. I stayed with Jorge every minute that I possibly could and on Sunday January 29, I came home.

An hour later, I got a call from one of my new colleagues at Broadway House. They wanted to be sure I was going to be back at work Monday morning because we were set to get our very first patient.

Jorge was hanging on in Puerto Rico. Ed was able to get a flight for Jorge from Puerto Rico to Newark so Jorge would have his wish to die in New Jersey. Ed called to let us know Jorge would be arriving at Newark Airport on Saturday, February 4. Pito, Jorge's dad, was coming with him and would stay at our house, which is walking distance to St. Francis Hospital. Ed would come later with Elsa, his and Jorge's mom. I called Jeff and Luis right away to ask if they would be able to help us out. Of course they agreed.

The plane arrived on schedule; Jorge was taken off the plane on a stretcher. Pito followed with a suitcase in his hand. We took Jorge directly to St. Francis and Dr. Mangia examined him. Jorge was happy to be back, but we could tell he was in pain. The lymphedema was spreading to the point where even his abdomen was swelling and the weight of the fluid was beginning to choke off his air supply.

We had to keep the head of the bed raised to 90 degrees the whole time. Once Jorge settled in, his nurses asked that we come back in the morning so they could do the tests and procedures they needed to do.

On Sunday, Pito went back to the hospital first thing in the morning. Bob and I went to church and asked the Ladies of Grace to pray for Jorge. They all knew him because he sometimes went to church with us.

After church, Bob and I stopped in to see Jorge and give Pito a break. He went to our house and what does he do? He cooks us a grand Sunday dinner Puerto Rican style. Jorge looked much more comfortable that day than when he arrived; the nurses did a fantastic job. They also had two reclining chairs next to Jorge's bed so that someone could be with him 24/7.

I called Joan Quigley the hospital's Vice President of Communications to let her know how pleased we were with the treatment Jorge was receiving. Joan was also our Assemblywoman and lived on the same block as my family when we lived on Fairmount Avenue. I am happy and proud to say I voted for her in every election. She is a wonderful human being.

We all knew the end was near for Jorge and the process now was to be sure he was as comfortable as possible, and to make sure his family and friends were all there. Most everyone who could be there was there and others who could not were in touch by phone. Food and drinks were available at our home thanks to Bob and Pito. Bob was always baking something and Pito was cooking meals for everyone.

During the day while I was at work tending to the new patients arriving at Broadway house, Pito and others were there for Jorge. In the evening, when I came home, I would eat dinner and shower, then head up to the hospital and stay until I couldn't keep my eyes open any more. Then I would go home to bed.

Jorge asked if we could get a cake to celebrate his brother's birthday, which we did. Barry, Jeff, Luis, Bob and I were all there. Shortly after his brother's birthday, Jorge had become aphasic and could only speak with his eyes.

For three days, all we could do was hold his hand and tell him we loved him and that it was going to be alright if he let go. Jorge could not respond.

## My Funny Valentine

It was February 14, Valentine's Day, the best day to tell or show someone how much you love them. We had the units at Broadway House decorated. I came home from work and after dinner I went to the hospital and sat in the recliner next to Pito, who was by Jorge's side the whole day.

Jorge was upright in bed and his breathing was very shallow; his eyes closed. He was very still, and I checked his pulse and respirations. In the eleven months that I knew Jorge he had become a very special friend to Bob and me, and brought much joy to our lives.

The time had come for Jorge. I stood next to his bed, fixed his hair, fluffed his pillow and stroked his hand. At about 9:15 pm, Jorge opened his eyes, and looked right at me, gasping for a last breath. He grabbed my hand and said, "I love you." I replied, "I love you, too, Jorge." Then he closed his eyes. I waited a few seconds to gather myself in disbelief of what had just happened. I wondered if people would believe me when I told them.

I shook Pito, who had been sleeping, and nodded my head "yes."

Pito wept. I left him alone with Jorge, called the nurse, and she confirmed and recorded Jorge's passing. Valentine's Day has always been my favorite holiday; it was now extra special.

It had been agreed earlier that Jorge's family would take him back to Puerto Rico for burial. Bob and I would not attend, as the family wanted a private ceremony for immediate family only.

We would hold a memorial service for Jorge in Jersey City at a later date, so his friends and family could attend.

After Jorge's family scattered his ashes in Puerto Rico, Bob and I received this letter from Jorge's brother Ed. He wrote,

*"Dear Dominick & Bob. We know that Jorge is in a much better place because of your kindness and attentions. You gave him real peace by the good things you did for him. Your thoughtfulness and care for Jorge, Mami and Papi, and my whole family are still very much in our minds. I hope these short lines can deliver the biggest and warmest thank you I can muster."*

Jorge's Memorial Service was held April 8 at Greenville Memorial Funeral Home. My life-long friend Lou Squitieri owns Greenville, and when Jorge died, I called Lou and told him about my plan to do a Memorial Service there. Lou not only said yes to that request, he had already helped Jorge's family take Jorge's ashes back to Puerto Rico. Lou is one of those friends who is always there for me. We may not see each other every day but we know we are just a phone call away. Lou was terrific with providing a space for Jorge's Memorial Service and he never asked me for a dime to do it.

## We'll Always Be Bosom Buddies

The first time I met Lou, I was engaged to be married, Lou, was also engaged. We were both 19 when me met. As Lou would put it now, "What were we thinking?"

Lou and I both have family members with Thalassemia, a blood disease that affects people of Mediterranean descent similar to Sickle Cell Anemia, which affects African-Americans. Sickle Cell Anemia is a disease that forces blood cells to become sickle shaped and cause blockages in blood vessels; it can be very painful. Thalassemia also causes blockages, but it causes the blood cells to become inflated, which can also be very painful.

Lou and I became volunteers for Cooley's Anemia Volunteers of New Jersey. When the call for volunteers for Cooley's Anemia was announced, many Italian-Americans showed up to volunteer; Lou and I were among the youngest ones there.

Lou is very Italian, dark hair, big nose and black dark-rimmed glasses. When we met, one of the first things he said to me was *"Hi, I'm Lou Squitieri and the answer is no! When I take off my glasses, my nose and moustache don't come with it."*

Lou said this when he wanted to loosen the mood. I liked him immediately.

We only saw each other at those meetings. Then he got married; I got married. We went our separate ways and led our separate lives, only seeing each other at occasional functions and fundraisers for Thalassemia.

We're both Italian, touchy-feely, warm and friendly guys, and at the time we both understood that we had to keep our friendship in tact while living our lives. There was something that drew us together, a feeling that our connection was going to be life-long.

One day I was on my way to my lawyer's office near Journal Square to sign my divorce papers. I'm crossing a busy intersection

98

when Lou pulls up in his car and calls out my name. We chatted for a few minutes, I told him where I was headed and he said: "I'm going through a separation, too. Here's my number, give me a call."

The next weekend, I called him and we got together for dinner. Lou told me all about his separation; I told him about what I was going through with my divorce. This is where we came out to each other.

Lou and I love each other very much, we are like Old Italian "aunties" and we have so much fun telling people that. Although we were both young, good-looking guys just coming out of the closet, and opportunities arose, we loved each other in a platonic way, and our friendship was always more important than anyone can imagine.

Lou was always very confident, compared to me. I tended to be unsure with the direction of my life. Not Lou. He knew he was going to be a successful mortician. At the time, we were two friends dealing with life in different ways. Sometimes I fed off his strength; and his ability to make me laugh about serious issues was a great relief.

Every encounter with Lou was like going to a comedy show. I always left feeling better than when I came in. He's just a really funny guy.

The Memorial Service Lou gave Jorge was a great tribute to Jorge, and his family and friends were all there. Robert Mason sang a few songs, and each person in attendance was asked to say a few words about how Jorge touched their lives. Many got up to speak. My friend Keith drew a picture of Jorge.

Lou was terrific and at the end of the Memorial Service, he lightened up the sadness in his usual style. He closed the ceremony by saying, "Dominick & Bob will be hosting everyone at their

home for a repast in Jorge's honor. Before he died, Jorge requested that a party be held for him, so when you get there, have fun
and Jorge will smile down on you. If you cry and don't have fun,
and Jorge were here, he'd say, *"You are evil and must be destroyed."*
And, for those of you who never met me, the answer is no! My
nose and mustache do not come off when I take off my glasses."

We got back to our house, and there was plenty of food and
music. We had balloons and party hats just like Jorge wanted and
everyone was talking, laughing, and honoring Jorge. Bob and I
ran around being the best party hosts we could and made sure
we took care of Jorge's family.

Later that day, Bob and I had just put our feet up and the
phone rang again. He said his name was Paul and that he was a
friend of Jorge's.

"Somebody told me he was living there," Paul said, "and I'd
like to speak to him, if he's there."

Paul and Jorge had met before Christmas and became
friends. I think they were interested in each other, but Jorge
didn't want to get close because he knew he wasn't going to be
around much longer.

I could feel the blood leave my head. "Um, where do you
live? Is it okay if I stop over?" I asked him. I didn't want to tell
Paul anything over the phone. He lived two blocks away on Jersey
Avenue and I told him I'd meet him in five minutes. He was sitting on his front steps when I arrived.

I could feel there was a real attachment between Paul and
Jorge and I knew I had to somehow find the strength to tell him
that Jorge had died. I took his hand, put my arm around him and
said, "I don't know how to tell you this, but we just had Jorge's
Memorial Service."

Paul broke down and cried right there on the steps. "Had I known about you, I would have called to invite you to his Memorial Service," I told him.

When Paul met Jorge it was shortly before he moved in with us. I don't think Jorge felt comfortable giving Paul our address and phone number. Of course if he had that would have been fine with us.

Paul and I got together a few times after that. I gave him pictures of Jorge, and a pair of boots Jorge owned that Paul really liked. I really wish that Jorge and Paul could have known each other longer; they would have made a beautiful couple.

# The White Tornado

During the six months that had passed since Jorge's death, my ability to learn more about the job was fair, at best. I had trouble concentrating and the loss of Jorge took its toll on me physically, emotionally and mentally. It had been only six months, and already I was feeling burned out. Much of it had to do with Michael Nelson, the Director of Nursing who hired me right on the spot, took the time to help me develop my skills, and then left abruptly, with no explanation. I was devastated.

There were rumors flying all over the place, but I chose not to believe any of them. I wanted to see him or talk to him myself, but he never responded to anyone's calls, cards, or letters. Meanwhile, many of my friends and patients were dying, and I was trying to keep it all together the best I could.

We were then introduced to the new Director of Nursing Mrs. B. The first thing she said to me was, "How long have you been a nurse?"

I told her I had just graduated from nursing school in June of 1994.

"Oh no! How could they make you the Assistant Head Nurse of a unit with no experience?" she said, and immediately demoted me to staff nurse. I was fine with it. I didn't lose any money, and I didn't have to work as hard as the charge nurse. And the 3-11 pm shift gave me the opportunity to care for the patients and meet their families.

Mrs. B verbally jabbed me every chance she got, and went over my work with a fine-tooth comb. She also wrote me up more times than necessary, I thought. The only reason she never fired me, I'm guessing, was because patients' families were sending letters to Broadway House thanking me for helping them through a difficult time. Some even came back to volunteer or make donations to Broadway House in memory of their loved ones. I'm pretty sure the care I gave had a lot to do with that, but it also seemed to have no affect on Mrs. B whose negative attitude toward me made it more and more difficult for me to do my job.

I thought back to Jorge. Caring for him taught me several things. When death is imminent, every patient deserves to die with dignity. I learned it is imperative that someone be present when a patient takes their last breath; and that the care I give every patient should be equal to, or better than, the care I gave Jorge.

# Four

## 1996
## H.E.L.P. is On the Way

One of our new residents I'm caring for at Broadway House is Lisa who became HIV-positive from IV drug use. Lisa is indirectly related to me; at the time I did not know this. Her family lives around the corner from Bob and me on Brunswick Street.

Lisa has a six year-old, Alex, and one Saturday, I was hanging an IV for Lisa. When I looked up, my cousin Sam and his wife Jane were standing in the doorway of her room. They knew I worked there, but I had no idea Lisa was Jane's niece.

My cousin Sam and I are not close in age, but we always had a good relationship. Sam and his brother Paul are always at the house on holidays and before I met Bob, Sam used to do my taxes. I was surprised to see them.

Strange, but shortly before that day, Lisa was in the activities room and drew me a picture with my initials made of flowers, and on the bottom she wrote *"To Dom, Love ya like Family."*

Because Lisa's mother, Betty works at Christ Hospital and lives nearby, we talk a lot. This one time, she says to me, "I wish Lisa had met you a long time ago. You may have been able to guide her in a different direction and find support for her."

Her words spark an idea I have been tossing around in my head lately. I've been thinking of starting an AIDS support group.

Betty tells me that support groups in Jersey City are not dealing with the issues affecting her daughter. Other people I ask say the same thing: support group facilitators do not always know how to help group members with HIV/AIDS get the social services they need. And since group facilitators are not always medical professionals, they cannot advise a group member on the best medical care. Sure, group members may have an opportunity to vent their issues, but they come back with the same unresolved issues week-after-week. I wanted to change that.

For this reason, while deciding to start an AIDS support group, I changed the word "support" to "empowerment" thereby giving members a support group where they can learn to advocate for themselves when it comes to medical attention and social services.

# Three Hugs a Day

It's February and we've been pelted with a huge snowstorm three days in a row and it has buried our area under almost 3 feet of snow. The nurses at Broadway House are called in; we were told on the phone to pack a bag with clothes for a few days. The National Guard picks me up in a huge camouflage army truck.

I spend a lot of time with the residents, staying up late, working two shifts because some nurses are not able to make it in. About a week goes by and the *Jersey Journal* sends a newspaper reporter and photographer to do a story on Broadway House.

One of the residents tells the reporter, Sally Deering, about my hug system: I give all residents, who want hugs, three huge hugs a day. One hug in the morning after rounds, one after lunch or when meds are passed out, and one before I leave to go home.

The story is published and it mentions that I will be starting a new empowerment group in Jersey City called, "PROJECT H.E.L.P. (Hugs Expressing Love of People living with HIV/AIDS). The group's meetings are to be held at Grace Lutheran Church in Jersey City – the church Bob and I attend.

So, it's official. I am now the leader of Project H.E.L.P., a support/empowerment group for people living with HIV/AIDS. I will soon have a new family of people to care for besides my patients at Broadway House.

# If You Build It They Will Come

When I was in nursing school, part of our Psych rotation was to facilitate a support group. I facilitated an AA (Alcoholics Anonymous) group and an NA (Narcotics Anonymous) group, a Hyacinth Foundation HIV/AIDS group, and a F.A.I.T.H. Services HIV/AIDS support group in Hoboken. These groups are where I would bring my HIV-positive friends to seek the help they needed.

The difference between Project H.E.L.P. and other groups would be a new concept called "Own Who You Are". This concept puts the responsibility of fundraising efforts on the members. No handouts. Instead, group members will feel a sense of accomplishment and belonging based on a shared desire to do good for the group. I also wanted to fund the group without asking for grant money from city, state or government sources like the Ryan White Care Act.

How can a support/empowerment group survive without funding from government sources or foundations? Most people don't know that once an organization is funded by money from the city, state or Ryan White Care Act, it has to prove its worth by way of numbers – number of group members must always increase; monies raised must match funding offered, and so on. Sooner or later, every non-profit support group has to compete with other groups for membership and the same funding dollars. To me, this seems counter-productive. A dollar falls on the ground and 50 people dive for it. You have to be extremely aggressive to get the prize and it becomes more about the money than helping people with HIV/AIDS.

I would start Project H.E.L.P. for people who have one goal in mind: to live the best lives they possibly could while living with HIV.

If they are trying to take care of themselves, and willing to participate and learn to be self-sufficient, then I say, "Come on in." Our mission statement is simple: "We help those who help themselves."

The group will always meet in a church because people need a safe space to share. We raise our own money of which almost 100% goes directly back to the group members. The staff is all volunteers, including me.

About a month before I started my group, I wrote a letter to my family and friends – about 300 letters went out. I asked them to consider a donation of any amount they could spare to help me get Project H.E. L. P. started. I received over $2,000.

I used my own money to help fix up the church basement. Church basements are not always kept very well, and this one had been underutilized for years. It had square floor tiles that popped up from the rain, and it desperately needed a paint job. So we started a Church Building Fund and fixed the floors, painted the walls, fixed up the stage and got the stage curtain to work so we could do variety shows to raise more money for the repairs. Also in the basement was a Sunday school room that wasn't being used anymore, so I painted it white with red trim, and laid down a carpet. We were ready to start for our first meeting of Project H.E.L.P.

# Big Girls Don't Cry

It is Monday, April 8, that Project H.E.L.P. holds its first meeting. We are to start at 7 o'clock. I get there early to make coffee and put out bottles of water, chocolate chip cookies, cheese and crackers. I put the chairs in a circle. Even if no one shows up, I think, I'll do it again next Monday. It just takes a little time.

Taking a line from the movie *Field of Dreams*, "If you build it, they will come." I know that whatever God has in mind for this group, I am prepared to carry out the task. This will surely be a wait-and-see situation. My faith tells me, God provides and never gives you more than you can endure. I'm nervous and optimistic.

At 6:30, the first person walks in, a tall woman with big brown eyes that smile when she smiles.

"Hi, my name is Florence Holmes." she says, "I'm not HIV positive, but I know a lot of people who are, and I'd like to help them. Can I volunteer?"

I invite her in and silently say, "Thank you God. You just plopped this amazing woman into my life. How lucky can I be?"

Florence and I talk and I share my vision for the group.

"That's incredible,' Florence says. "That's exactly what I was hoping it would be. I know people in my neighborhood who are living with this virus and I plan to bring them to group. I wanted to scope it out first to see if we were on the same page."

The next person that walks in is Roro, a petite brunette with big brown eyes. She says, "Hi, is this where the support group meets?"

107

I nod "yes" and invite her in.

Roro says, "I read an article in the *Jersey Journal* about this new group and since I live just a few blocks away, I thought I'd come by to see what it's about. My fiancé just died and I don't really know what to do next?"

I offer Roro a seat and Florence brings her a bottle of water and a plate of goodies. We chat and wait to see if anyone else shows up. The pastor stops by to see how everything is going. I invite him to stay in case anyone has spiritual needs he can address.

I start the meeting by introducing myself and telling everyone why I felt the need to start the group. The pastor welcomes everyone and tells us he's available for spiritual support. Then Florence talks about how she's affected and how people she knows and loves are infected. She wants to learn more and help more. This was the most giving woman I had ever met.

We open the floor to Roro, who says she feels very comfortable after Florence and I welcomed her. As an activist I have heard many horrifying stories of young gay men being excommunicated from their church, disowned by their families, fired from their jobs, evicted from their apartments, tossed out of hospitals, shunned by their life partners, beaten, and even murdered for being gay and or having AIDS. I thought there was nothing else to know about the pain of living with HIV; until I listened to Roro.

"I grew up in New York and moved to New Jersey when I got married," Roro begins. "I got a divorce from my husband and we have a son who lives with his father. I hardly see him or speak with him."

My boyfriend, Gerald and I were living here in Jersey City and me, "I'm a sunshine girl," I love the beach. Gerald and I always had a dream to move to Florida and live under a palm tree. I'm a waitress, so I can work anywhere.

About a year ago, we do it, Gerald and I move to Florida and we're ready to live our dream: get married, have a baby and just be happy. After we make the move, I start feeling sick every day and it turns out, I'm pregnant. We aren't married yet but when I find out I'm pregnant, we decide to marry right away. I go for the blood test and the doctor tells me to come see him. I sit in the exam room and he tells me I have AIDS. I just couldn't believe it. I mean, I'm a good girl. I don't do drugs, and I don't fool around, I'm a good girl."

"Go on." I say, putting my arm around her for support.

"The doctor told me I have to decide what to do about the pregnancy. I can't believe what I'm hearing! He also tells me Gerald has to come in and be tested. He did the next day and was diagnosed with AIDS too. So here we are in Florida, our dream turned into a nightmare.

I didn't know if I should keep the baby or have an abortion, and I didn't know where else to turn, or what else to do.

"Gerald decided he was not going to take the prescribed medication. I wanted to take it. I am a fighter and I want to live. Knowing that, I also did not want to be alone, in Florida, with a baby with AIDS, not knowing how long I would have to live to take care of her. I had to terminate my pregnancy. They told me my baby was a girl. I named her Melissa Kate.

"Gerald didn't make it. He got sick very quickly and died. All I was left with was a broken dream, so I moved back to Jersey City, found myself a new job and now I am out of medication and looking for help. When I saw the article about you and Project H.E.L.P., I knew I had to be here tonight."

Roro turns to the pastor and says, "I was raised Catholic, but I have not been to church in a long time. Is it okay if I come to church here on Sunday? I really need God in my life."

The pastor says, "Yes, of course you can, and you can call on me anytime if you need to talk."

Florence chimes in saying, "Here is my number, too, I love to cook, so if you need food or you just want company, give me a call."

As an AIDS Nurse, my immediate concern for Roro is getting her into care right away. I give her my phone number, and set her up with an appointment at F.A.I.T.H. Services in Hoboken. I also give her the number for the Hyacinth Foundation in New Brunswick. In the weeks to come, when her doctor prescribes a triple drug therapy that includes Crixivan. I set her up with a payment plan through my friend Sandra, a nurse and representative for Merck pharmaceuticals. Sandra puts Roro on the free Patient Assistance program.

At the end of the meeting we all stand up and hold hands in a circle, a ritual done at every other support group meeting I've attended. We say a little prayer of thanks to God for bringing us together. Florence helps me clean up the kitchen. I hug her three times and say "thank you so much; you are a blessing to me."

"No! Thank you," Florence says. "The blessing is you for starting this group. You have already helped the world become a better place. I will be back next week. I want to be a part of this incredible project."

## Whispers of Concern

The following week a handsome young man, Dan, in his 20s, arrives with his mother, Cheryl.

She pulls me aside and whispers, "my son's not homosexual, he is a hemophiliac."

"I'll take very good care of him," I tell her. "Would you like to stay?"

"No, he doesn't want me to; I just wanted to let you know that," she says.

I give her a big hug, thank her, and tell her it will be okay.

Before 1985, many hemophiliacs received blood transfusions infused with blood that was not tested and thousands became infected with HIV. Dan was just a young boy like Ryan White when he received his transfusion. I can't even imagine how he, his mother, and family felt that day when they found out, nor can I imaging having to be the medical professional who told them. In 1985, it was written into law that all donated blood products have to be tested for HIV.

I totally understood what Cheryl meant when she pointed out that Dan wasn't homosexual. It seems Dan had tried other HIV/AIDS support groups, but the gay men that attended, many of them chased after Dan for a date. I don't judge that to be dirty or harassing. You see, when a person is diagnosed with HIV/AIDS one of the first thoughts they have – after the initial shock – is, who will love me now that I'm sick? Many go to support groups to meet someone also living with HIV, someone who understands what it's like.

Dan was pretty quiet most of the meeting and when it was his turn to speak he addressed the issue his mother spoke to me about. He said he felt comfortable because the only other group member was Roro, a woman.

During the past week, Roro said she had her best week in a long time. She felt very secure with her new doctors and nurses at St. Mary Hospital and the social workers at F.A.I.T.H. Services. She also attended church at Grace Lutheran the day before the second group meeting and she felt the warm embrace of a most loving and caring group of congregants. Roro expressed her appreciation that put a smile on all of our faces. She did have only one issue she wanted to talk about: the pills.

Roro is taking the triple-drug therapy, which means she has to swallow 15 pills a day. We make a point of saying, every dose, on time, every day. Roro doesn't like it, but she does it.

I remember one night being awakened by the telephone at 11:30. It was Roro in a panic. "I came home from work and fell asleep," she says. "My 10 pm pills, I didn't take them and it's 11:30. Am I going to get sick now? "

I reassure her that if she takes her 10 pm a little late, she will not get sick.

"Take them now and I will call you tomorrow and check up on you," I tell her.

She hangs up, relieved.

The next day I check on her and she keeps apologizing for waking me. I tell her, "No worries. I would rather you call me when you are not sure, you did the right thing."

That week between the first and second group I put together a Board of Directors. I will lead the group meetings, and do the fundraising plan; Bob will perform secretarial duties; Robert Mason is in charge of the money and opened an account for the group at Provident Bank where he's a Vice President, and Florence will be in charge of volunteers.

For the next few weeks it's just Roro and Dan. While a lot is accomplished, I'm hoping more people will show up. Word about the group needed time to circulate. I had to learn patience. "If you build it they will come, right?"

Because of Project H.E.L.P. and the networking systems that were being organized, I began to broaden my horizons by attending all sorts of events and meetings that were going on throughout New Jersey. I began to meet people who, like me, provided a variety of services to the population we served.

It's mid-July and I attend a meeting of the Ryan White Community Outreach and Support Center in South Orange, New Jersey. At this meeting I meet several representatives from other AIDS Service Organizations (ASO's) in New Jersey. I came to represent Project H.E.L.P. of course. Each representative was invited to stand up and explain the services their organization provides.

When I tell the group that Project H.E.L.P. is more of an empowerment group than a support group, they seem to be impressed by the concept. Three days later I receive a personal letter from Quintin John Clough, MSW, and director Matthew Colacurto. They connect me with AIDS-Line, a monthly publication of all the services available in the State and they refer one of their clients to Project H.E.L.P.

As word spreads about Project H.E.L.P., new members are joining all the time. I'm asked by Rev. Bruce Davidson to become a member of the "Lutheran AIDS Task Force" and I even give a speech at the Synod Assembly. Roro is on her new medications for only a month and at group she announces her T-cell count went up and her viral load is undetectable.

In August, we support volunteer Ricardo, who is bicycling in the Boston-to-New York AIDS Ride. He needs to raise $1500 to participate and Project H.E.L.P. and Grace Church help him raise over $200 of it. The summer ends with a BBQ at our home in Jersey City.

We have a new extended family, our Project H.E.L.P. family: Roro, Florence, Dan, and all our new members, each one with a

Dominick P Varsalone and Sally Deering

unique story to share. Of course, I can't leave out my Italian family. In fact, Bob and I live just a few blocks from my childhood home on Montgomery Street, where I first found out I was different from the rest of my family.

# 1956
## Mi Famiglia

I come from a strict Italian family, a Baby Boomer baby near the end of a line of eight kids growing up in Jersey City, New Jersey in the late 1950s. There were 11 of us in all: my mother, who was a stay-at-home mom; dad, a freight train repairman; my two adopted brothers, Gilbert; and Johnny, (who only lived with us for a short time) and my older adopted sister, Veronica. There were my two older biological sisters, Alice and Susan, and my older biological brother Salvatore, then me. I was born on Mother's Day, Sunday May 13, 1956. My younger sister, Mary Jo, arrived almost four years after me in 1960. With Grandma, it added up to eleven people cramped in a seven-room apartment surviving on my father's salary as a railroad train repairman.

My three adopted siblings; John, Gilbert and Veronica are actually my cousins, the children of my mother's older sister, Florence. We were told that at 35, Aunt Florence's husband died suddenly from a massive heart-attack and shortly after, Aunt Florence had a nervous breakdown, couldn't handle three children, and they institutionalized her.

John, Gilbert and Veronica (we called her Mary) were 19, 17, and 5 at the time, and they might know the story a little differently. I say this because in many Italian families back then, parents hid the real truth, especially when there was a sticky family issue

114

to handle. Instead of telling what really happened, they buried the truth and made something up that sounded plausible.

After becoming a nurse, I learned that some of our family stories were fabricated and much more dramatic than what we were told.

It was rumored by some that Aunt Florence actually killed her husband, and for reason of insanity, was placed in a psychiatric facility instead of prison. Is this true? Who knows? Aunt Florence was committed to a mental institution in Secaucus, the same place my grandfather committed Uncle Mickey some years earlier.

Back then, our parents told us kids that Aunt Florence had a nervous breakdown because she couldn't handle her husband's death and then have the wherewithal to raise three kids. Who were we to question anything our parents told us; we took all they said as the truth. Dad was a master at fabricating stories and mom would always go along because wives did as they were told back then and did not question their husbands.

During the first years of my parents' marriage, my mother had four miscarriages and the doctors back in the mid-1940's said she'd never be able to have children, so, my parents legally adopted John, Gilbert and Veronica. Shortly after adopting my cousins my parents went on to have five children of their own, despite the odds the doctors had given.

# Love Hurts

When my grandfather committed his son, my Uncle Mickey, to an institution, they said it was because Uncle Mickey had brain damage. That wasn't true.

The story goes that months away from his high school graduation, Uncle Mickey got into a fight with some boy over a girl and the boy pushed Uncle Mickey down a flight of stairs. I was just a kid when my parents told me. They said Uncle Mickey hit his head on the cement steps and was never the same. That's what they told me, and it wasn't until many years later that I learned what really happened.

After my father retired, and my parents moved from New Jersey to Florida, they made me Uncle Mickey's "Caretaker Proxy" that gave me Power of Attorney, and I would visit him at the institution.

During one of my visits, I met his social worker. We talked and during our conversation, I asked her about Uncle Mickey's admitting diagnosis. The social worker told me according to the *Diagnostic and Statistical Manual of Mental Health Disorders, No. 1,"* (DSM-1,) Uncle Mickey had been admitted for homosexuality.

I was floored. I just sat there, stunned. Right then and there, I realized not everything my family told me was the whole truth. They concocted the whole story about him having a fight over a girl, hitting his head and then being brain-damaged. The truth was that his own father committed him because he was a gay boy. They took him out of high school, never even let him graduate or go to his prom and put him in a mental institution because he and another boy felt a spark for each other.

I went home that night and did some research. Sure enough, according to the DSM-1, published in 1952, homosexuality was a mental health diagnosis. It was also a mental health diagnosis in the DSM-2 published in 1968. This did not change until 1973 when the Board of Trustees of the American Psychiatric Association (APA) voted to eliminate the category of "Homosexuality" and replace it with "Sexual Orientation Disturbance". The DSM-3, which was published in 1980, reflected this change.

So, they changed it from "psychotic homo", to "sexually disturbed homo"? Actually, the APA decided to rewrite it because so few psychiatrists used the DSM-1 & 2 mental health diagnosis.

During Uncle Mickey's time in the institution, which spanned almost 70 years, the doctors performed Electric Shock Therapy (ECT) treatments on him to "cure" him of his homosexuality. As part of his treatment, they gave him psychotropic medications, which caused him to become a mental vegetable. Psychotropic medications are given for people with an imbalance in their brain and if those drugs are given to someone who does not have that brain imbalance it can be very harmful, which certainly was the case for Uncle Mickey.

When I was a child, I used to go with my grandma to visit him. She would bring him baked ziti, spaghetti and meatballs, and hamburgers and I would go along for the ride to keep her company. It was usually Uncle Vincent who drove but if he could not make it we would take the bus together.

We would go to Uncle Mickey's room or the large visitor's community room and sit with him. The only thing Uncle Mickey could say was my name. I often wonder today if he resented me because my parents named me after his father who committed him. He also memorized everyone's birthday in the family. He memorized his brothers', sisters' and mother's birthday; everyone except his father. He never talked about him. It's really funny because of all my siblings, I am the one most likely to remember a birthday and send a card to everyone in the family and to special friends.

I now believe my grandmother and grandfather divorced because of Uncle Mickey's situation (of course that was kept all hush-hush as well). I'm not certain they actually went through an official divorce or if grandma just moved out. I am sure she didn't want her son committed because of his sexuality. My sainted grandmother who I loved probably never understood it, though I am certain it hurt her deeply. And although it all happened before I was born, I'm sure that's how she came to live with us.

And that's how I learned my family's confusing attitudes about homosexuality. I couldn't verbalize it to myself at the time, but looking back, there must have been a part of me that assumed that if my parents ever thought I was a homosexual, they'd commit me to an insane asylum, like grandpa did to Uncle Mickey. The only person I knew I could tell was my grandmother. Somehow I knew, even back then, that if I told her I was gay, she'd love me anyway.

This is the reason I feel my grandmother knew my sexuality during my early years and this is why she was so protective of me. I was most definitely her favorite grandchild, which was important to me because I never felt that kind of love from anyone else in my family, especially not my father or brother.

Don't get me wrong. I always knew they loved me, but they never made it known publicly or did it out loud in front of others. I listen to young fathers today who call their little boys "buddy". It makes me think more of my first dog than something my dad would call me.

My dad was a freight train repairman for the Penn Central Railroad in Kearny, New Jersey. He did that all of his working life; 40 years, and he supported eleven people on his salary. I still don't know how he did it, but I guess it wasn't so bad back then. As kids, we didn't have much, but our needs were taken care of somehow. I always heard people say my grandmother and my mom could turn dimes into dollars.

On dad's pay day, we would wait for him to come home and he would give each of us a quarter allowance, and we ran to the corner store for penny candy. It seemed like that little brown paper sack would be filled to the top with goodies that we would make last the whole week.

## Goombahs Go Gaelic

We lived in a 7-room apartment on the third floor of 326 Montgomery Street, an orange brick, four-family building in the downtown section of Jersey City known as "Van-Vorst." Montgomery Street is one of Jersey City's main streets and from our apartment, if you walked east about a half-mile, you would be at the Hudson River waterfront facing the New York City Skyline.

This area of Jersey City is the city's most historic because it was the first to be populated by the Dutch, the earliest settlers of Jersey City and the same folks who bought Manhattan Island from the Native Americans. Later on, several European cultures – German, Italian, Irish, Jewish – settled in different sections known as Downtown, the Village (where we lived), Marion, the Heights, Journal Square, and Bergen-Lafayette. And every section had its own Catholic parish. Little Italy was in the Village section where our family had settled, so we were members of Holy Rosary parish. When we lived in the Irish part of town, I attended St. Bridget's.

I remember our apartment. There was a 50-foot hall that went from one end to the other and all the rooms were off to the side. They called these "railroad rooms." I remember we always had a dog. Our first one was "Queenie". If I had known then what I know now, I would say they named the dog after me. Go figure.

At 326 Montgomery Street, in the long hallway that ran throughout the apartment, my brother Sal would set up his toy army soldiers and then tell me I couldn't play with him. So I would wait until he had them all set up and then throw something to knock them down. This would make him mad and he would call me all sorts of names: sissy, Mary, faggot and queer were the most hurtful slangs back then. I have been called all of them.

My childhood was pretty good for the most part. We were a big Italian family and there was always a lot of yelling and always a lot of visitors, especially on holidays. Mom's brothers, sisters, aunts, uncles and cousins all came to our house, so they could see Grandma; and we always went to 333 Fifth Street to see Dad's side of the family.

After dinner, Mom's family would be in the kitchen playing cards or pokino. The kids would play board games, air hockey, and that soccer game with metal rods you turn to get the ball in the goal. I was never good at this game and never got to play it, either, except when my brother Sal wanted to play against someone he knew he could beat. I liked playing school and I was always the teacher with Mary Jo, Janine and Michelle as my students.

# 1972
## My Aunt Sadie Loved a Lady

My favorite aunt on my mother's side was Aunt Sadie, my mother's younger sister. Aunt Sadie never married, although my parents told us Aunt Sadie was engaged once. They told us the boy broke off the engagement, so Aunt Sadie turned her back on love, grew fat and took a job at Dixon Mills pencil factory in Jersey City.

Aunt Sadie was not an aunt we saw frequently. After she left her job at the pencil factory, which was before my time, she rarely left her apartment, a first-floor dilapidated place in a run-down apartment building on First and Monmouth Streets in Jersey City. She lived there with her friend, Jenny. I don't remember ever going inside. My older siblings seemed to know her far better than I did, but I think I got to know her better in the years just before Jenny's untimely death.

Jenny was a tall, thin woman with long gray hair that almost looked blonde. She must have been very beautiful in her day. I think Jenny was older than Sadie.

If you ask my older siblings, they'll tell you it was a matter of convenience that Jenny took care of Sadie and helped her as she did. But I think there might have been more than a friendship between the two women. I guess the only people who could describe their relationship were the two of them. Whatever they were to each other is between them and God.

Their relationship was very deep. I now think perhaps Aunt Sadie was a lesbian and knowing what happened to her brother Mike (Uncle Mickey), she was never able to live life out in the open. My vague memories of Jenny and Sadie together tell me they really did love each other. Gay or straight, there was something special there.

Aunt Sadie never brought Jenny to any of our family's holiday dinners and the only time I really saw them together was through their front window where Aunt Sadie would spend her time, leaning on the windowsill talking to neighbors and watching the world go by. Jenny was always inside, probably in the kitchen.

"Kid, would you buy me a quart of milk," she would say to some boy or girl hanging out on the sidewalk. Jenny was probably the one who took care of the apartment. Aunt Sadie didn't clean or cook or do any of those things.

She was kind and generous, sweet and soft-spoken. For going to the store she would give the kids pencils, hard candy and cash. She was not at all a combative or angry type of person, Aunt Sadie seemed happy in her little world with the few possessions she owned. Life was just what she wanted it to be – happy and content and very private. She was always smiling.

Jenny died in the 1960s and I have no idea from what. I don't remember her funeral or anybody talking about it. It was all hush-hush. After Jenny died, people would bring Sadie food or just stop by to check in on her to be sure she was okay. The inside of the apartment began to turn shabby from neglect. Aunt Sadie was a wonderful woman, but she was no housekeeper.

The apartment building Aunt Sadie lived in was actually connected to two other apartment buildings, one on each side. Some years after Jenny died, the City condemned all three build-ings and planned to raze them to the ground. They had big or-ange signs that read "Building Condemned" posted on the front doors.

By this time, it was 1972. All the other tenants had vacated their apartments except for Aunt Sadie. She was the only one who refused to leave her apartment – and the only one left. Inspectors would come to her building and she wouldn't let them into her apartment. She would slam the window down and tell them to go away. They even turned off her electricity in an effort to get her out and still, she wouldn't budge.

This was where she lived with her beloved friend Jenny. She couldn't bear the thought of leaving. If you ask me, Aunt Sadie wanted to die there.

Early one morning around this time, I answered the phone. It was Mom's brother, my Uncle Vincent. He tells me to put my mother on the phone; it's urgent. My mother grabs the phone.

"Vincent?"

"It's Sadie. She won't leave the house."

"What else is new?"

"There's no time left. The whole city of Jersey City is camped out in front of her building and she won't come out. The cops just called and they want us to go over there and get her out. I'll pick you up on the way; be ready."

And with that, he hung up and we were off to save Aunt Sadie from demolition. We piled into his car and headed over to Aunt Sadie's building. I am not certain why my mother made me come along. When we got there, it was just like Uncle Vincent described. Ambulances, fire trucks and police cars lined the streets outside the condemned building and cops were everywhere.

Neighbors had spilled out onto the streets and some in the apartments across the street were hanging out their windows to watch the show that was taking place below.

The day had come to tear the buildings down and Aunt Sadie wasn't budging.

One cop was yelling into a bullhorn when we pulled up to the tall redbrick building.

"Miss Sadie, you are in great danger. You must vacate the apartment and get out of the building NOW."

His voice sounded loud and desperate.

Silence.

"Miss Sadie. We will have to arrest you, and we will press charges."

Silence.

"Miss Montecalvo, please come out now," he begged and pleaded.

I'm sure if she were a frail old woman, they would have restrained her and hauled her out of there. This woman who I never heard say a curse word in her life, came to the window and yelled: "*Stunad! Sfacimm! Baffangul!*"

"Miss Sadie, please be reasonable. There's no more time left. You must leave the premises."

"*Vafanabola!*" Aunt Sadie called back. "You bunch of *finocchios.*"

They asked us to go in and talk her out. We went inside cautiously. Everything was dark and smelly. When we entered the apartment, the electricity was off, I am guessing it had been off for a while. We stood in the kitchen and there was Aunt Sadie at the kitchen table, holding a jewelry box that Jenny had given her.

"Sadie, it's time," my mother said, very softly.

"No, I won't go. They can't make me."

Then she pulls out this huge butcher knife.

"I'd rather stab myself in the heart with this knife than go,"

"You can't go on living like this. No electric. No gas. No water. I wouldn't let an animal live like this," my mother said.

"What am I going to do? Where am I going to go?" Aunt Sadie whimpered.

"We'll take care of you. You'll come and live with us. Then, when you're feeling better, we'll find you a nice apartment close by. Come on, Sadie."

Aunt Sadie sat there at the kitchen table crying while my mother collected her things.

"Here, put this in the car," she said, handing me suitcases filled with clothes and photographs. When my mother decided it was enough, she went over to Aunt Sadie and said, "Come on, Sadie, it's time."

We each got on either side of Aunt Sadie and helped her out of the chair. She kept clinging to the jewelry box.

"Let Dominick carry that," my mother said.

"NO!"

"Alright, alright, come on. Vincent is outside waiting with the car."

We walked Aunt Sadie through the crowd of cops, firefighters and construction workers and helped her into the front seat. We drove away, nobody saying a word. We walked out of there with our heads down as if we were criminals, the crowd outside was cheering and crying at the same time. The building demolition began as soon as we drove away. The next time I went down town it had become an empty lot, much like Sadie's life once Jenny was gone.

After about four months of living with us on West Side Avenue, Aunt Sadie moved into a nice first floor apartment on New York Avenue in the Heights. I would visit her occasionally and ask if she needed any help, but mostly it was to go to the store because she did not like going out of the house much.

Aunt Sadie weighed about 400 pounds at this point, and I think it was her extreme weight that made her a recluse. When no one was around to go to the store for her, Aunt Sadie sometimes ventured outside. It was during one of these times that she crossed the street between two parked cars, and was struck down by a car. She died a week later from pneumonia.

We later learned that the driver of the car told the policeman taking the report, "I did not see her crossing between those two parked cars." And the cop said, "WHAT DO YOU MEAN YOU DIDN'T SEE HER?"

There were no lawsuits or charges pressed.

It was the saddest funeral. Aunt Sadie was laid out at Intracasso & Angelo funeral home in Downtown Jersey City. In Italian culture, it's typical to become dramatic, emotional, even hysterical at a Wake. In order to get people to cry, funeral directors, especially those whose clients are Italian; hired women known as "professional criers." The criers wore black dresses and sat in the back of the funeral home and cried. They always wore black veils so you couldn't see their faces.

There were no professional criers at Aunt Sadie's funeral. I am guessing that there was no need, because her family was there, and more important, many of Aunt Sadie's neighbors came to pay their respects They all had stories about how she helped them one way or another. One of the young men who went to the store for her as a boy credited Aunt Sadie for putting him on the right path in life. I always ask myself why it is that we have to wait until a person dies to find out how wonderful they were to everyone who knew them.

I will never forget you, dear Aunt Sadie.

## *Scenes from my Scrapbook*

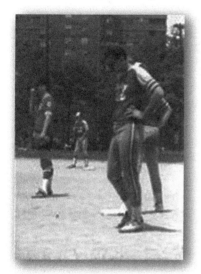

Man on first

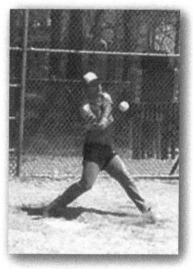

Batter up

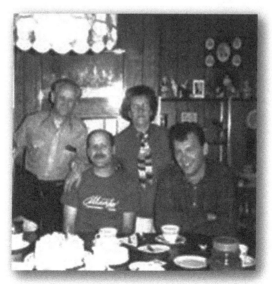

First date (Mother's Day 1986)

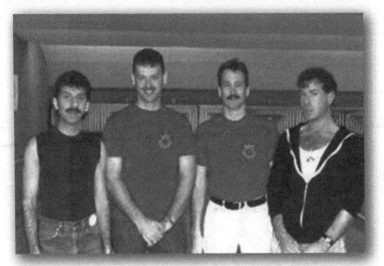

The bowling buds

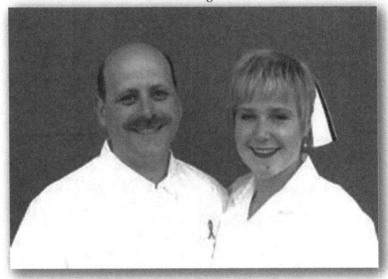

Doreen and I (Graduation 1994)

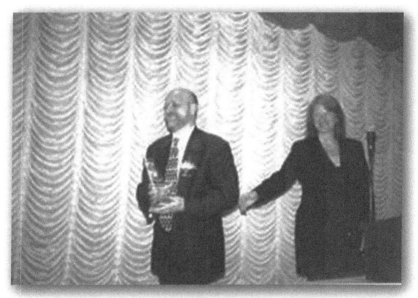

Everyday Hero award

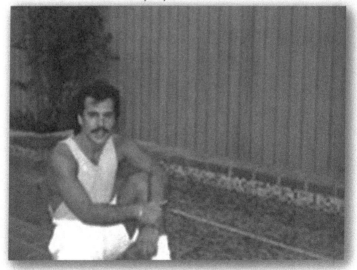

Jorge.

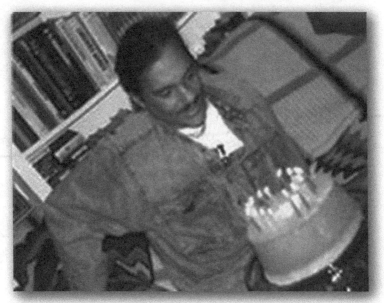

Jorge's birthday                    1995

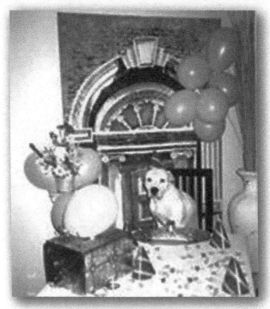

Ruffie's birthday

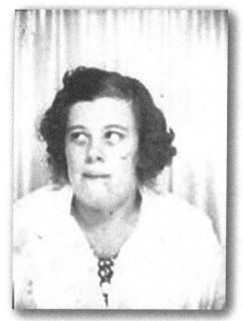

Aunt Sadie (circa 1950)

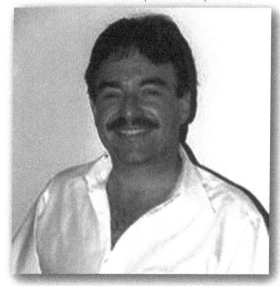

Lou Squitieri

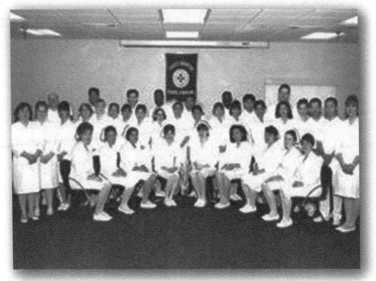

Graduation Class of 1994

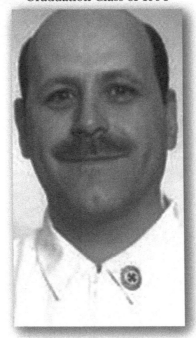

The Graduate

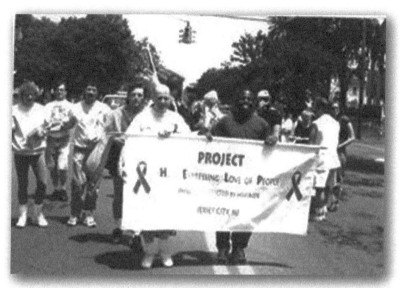

Project H.E.L.P. on Parade

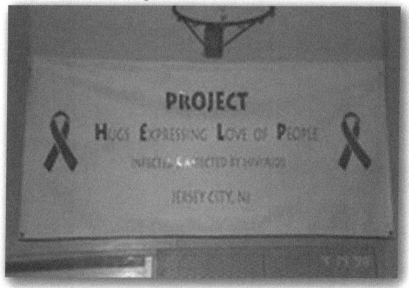

Project H.E.L.P. Banner

# Five

## 1997
## Promise Kept

Something is happening at Broadway House. Mrs. B. is making changes and everyone is being moved around to other units. I am just getting used to One East and Mrs. B switches me to Two East. Some nurses are getting promotions; others are being let go. This Director of Nursing is firing people for simple mistakes. Sometimes, nurses make errors, or poor decisions, but she has zero tolerance for those she doesn't like. The nurses she does like get the benefits.

Because I am one of the nurses that she doesn't like, I have to leave One East where I was caring for a very ill patient, Andy. I decided to place him in the same room with Edgar because Andy seemed to be giving up, even with his partner visiting him every day. I thought putting Andy with Edgar could inspire Andy to keep fighting. It was working for a while.

On Two East my job as charge nurse is becoming difficult. The LPN I'm assigned to work with is older and very tough. She pulls rank on me because of her nursing experience. What she doesn't realize is that while she has years of nursing experience, I have been a nurse in AIDS Care since the day I started my job and I was trained by Mike Nelson, the Director of Nursing at Broadway House; Carol O'Neil, the Assistant Director of Nursing; and Nancy Scangarello, a nurse at St. Michael's Medical Center who worked with Dr. George Perez, Director of Infectious Disease. This was the team that opened the first AIDS Clinic in Newark; and they were pioneers in their field.

The two CNAs I work with are nothing like Theresa and Beverly on One East and I struggle to get anyone to listen to me or do their job. Mrs. B tells me I don't have what it takes to be a Charge Nurse.

My residents on Two East are put upstairs on the second floor because they are more mobile than those on the first floor, which makes a lot of sense. Most of these patients are triple diagnosis: patients who have AIDS, substance abuse issues and mental health issues. My new assistant charge nurse calls them "The walkie-talkie trouble makers". I don't think its funny, but others seem to think it is.

On One East, two of the patients in my previous unit die five days apart: Shondra who had the most beautiful eyes; and Andy, Edgar's roommate. Edgar is extremely upset to lose his roommate, so I go downstairs to talk with him. He does really well walking with a cane, which most times he doesn't need. I remind him of the promise I made, a trip to the Gay Pride Parade in New York, which is just a week away. Employees are not allowed to take residents out on pass, but you know me, always trying to adjust the rules.

I go to Mrs. B. and she flat out refuses to let Edgar go with me to the Gay Pride Parade, so I go over her head to Mr. D, the Executive Director, who also says no. I have to keep my promise to Edgar somehow, so I call his sister and ask if she would sign him out for the day for a family outing and she does. It turned out to be one of the happiest days of Edgar's young life.

She comes early in the morning and signs him out from 8 am-to-8 pm. I meet them in Newark and take Edgar to church with me at Grace Lutheran in Jersey City and then we go to the Gay Pride Parade in New York. I carry a folding chair, speak to a policeman on the corner of 14th Street and 5th Avenue, and ask if Edgar can sit in front of the police barrier. I explain the situation and Edgar and I have front row seats for the whole parade.

Afterwards, I take him to dinner and sign him back into Broadway House. When Mrs. B finds out she goes ballistic on me.

Rumors spread about Edgar and me becoming "too chummy". My work at Broadway House is becoming more and more difficult, and I begin looking for a new job. I know and God knows, Edgar and I were not being "chummy," I was just fulfilling a promise.

All types of nursing jobs are available to me. Quite honestly I think I'm becoming depressed with all the death that has surrounded me as an AIDS Nurse. Now that there are medications prolonging peoples' lives, I want to work in a setting where I can educate my patients and empower them to thrive both physically and socially. I want to help crush the stigmas that came with an AIDS diagnosis. This is exactly what Project H.E.L.P. is all about.

It's Monday, August 12, and I walk into Mrs. B's office and give my two weeks notice to take a job at Newark Beth Israel Medical Center, right in the heart of Newark, which has one of the highest cases of HIV/AIDS in New Jersey. That is where the biggest need for my skills happens to be. Sure, I can take a job in New York City, caring for gay, white male patients, and making a much higher salary, but I already tend to that population with my friends. They all know I'm only a phone call away. I want to roll up my sleeves and be there for the people most ostracized and alienated.

In my last two weeks at Broadway House, I tell every resident where I'm going. I encourage them to strive for wellness and then come see me at the clinic for the continuation of their care.

As for Edgar, I speak with him and his sister and invite them both to come to a Project H.E.L.P. meeting any Monday they like. "Baby Boy" Edgar is Broadway House's biggest success story. Given two weeks to live, he made the decision to live and we (all the staff) made the care plan to pull off that miracle. I am so proud of him for fighting back against the AIDS Virus.

# Learning to Live Again

My new job as Staff Nurse at the Out-Patient Department, Infectious Disease Clinic at Newark Beth Israel Medical Center is a big change from Broadway House. I begin by preparing charts the day before clinic, making sure the most recent lab work is done and entered on the appropriate forms. On clinic day, I go from the office and walk across the street to the clinic with the charts in the order of the scheduled appointments. We see patients from 8:30 am until about noon, have our lunch, and then complete the paperwork from the office by calling in prescriptions for patients and doing follow-ups on their medical appointments. These assignments can sometimes be very involved and tedious, but most often we all pitch in and get the job done. Afterwards we continue the routine and prepare charts for the next clinic day.

There are three adult clinics per week for men and women run by the Medical Director, two pediatric clinics run by Dr. Mendelsohn and a woman's clinic run by Dr. Mammen Prasad. I am assigned to work the three adult clinics. Dr. Prasad did not want a male nurse to work the women's clinic at first and I did not want to work in Pediatric AIDS for fear of bringing home babies and small children to care for in my home and risk Bob filing for a divorce.

I occasionally help with the pre-clinic paperwork and fill in at the other clinics when a nurse is out sick or on vacation. I enjoy every aspect of all three clinics and quickly begin to fit right in with both my colleagues and the patients we treat. What is most rewarding about this job is that instead of holding a resident's hand and watching him or her die, I am learning a team approach to patient care and more often then not, I watch the patients thrive. Both are very important duties of an AIDS Nurse.

At Newark Beth Israel, one of the pediatric nurses left so I am asked to cover for her clinics while they search for a nurse with pediatric AIDS experience. I once said I would never work in pediatric AIDS, but here I am. Sometimes you just have to roll up your sleeves and work where the need is.

As it turns out, it is not terrible. I absolutely adore the babies and children and don't feel compelled to bring them all home to meet Bob.

My patient today is Colleen. I think she is about eight years old. Colleen is on a medication called Norvir. In its pill form it's very hard to swallow but it is being dispensed for a short time in liquid form only. Colleen is a trouper. Both her parents died from AIDS, so Colleen's grandmother takes care of her. On this particular visit, I call them into the next available exam room and do my usual routine duties and make conversation by asking questions about how everything has gone since their last visit. Colleen's grandmother says, "Nurse Dominick, maybe you can convince Colleen why she needs to take all of her medications."

I see Colleen sitting on the exam table pouting with her arms folded over her chest. This is a very unusual vibe I'm getting from both Colleen and Grandma. One is angry and the other stubborn, not the usual happy duo maintaining Colleen's health.

"Colleen, that's not like you," I tell her. "I know you always take your meds; you are a role model for other kids your age. What's going on?"

Colleen gives me a stone cold look and asks, "Have you ever tasted liquid Norvir, Nurse Dominick?"

I'm speechless for a second.

"No Colleen, I have never tasted liquid Norvir," I tell her.

"Well," she says, "it tastes like shit."

Grandma scolds Colleen and I bite my lower lip to maintain my professionalism and try not to burst into laughter. I reach over to pick up the bottle of liquid Norvir from the doctor's table. I open the cap and dab my pinky finger in and put the smallest amount of liquid Norvir possible on my pinky and taste it.

"Oh God, she's right," I tell them, "it tastes like shit."

After I finish the paperwork, I tell Grandma to go to the store and buy peanut butter and nutella when you go home. I carefully explain to Colleen that she should try each one separately. First she should try one teaspoon of peanut butter, then the liquid Norvir and then another teaspoon of peanut butter. At this point Colleen tells me she likes peanut butter almost as much as the liquid Norvir but she has never tasted nutella. I ask if she likes chocolate! Her reply, "Who doesn't?"

A month later we had the results of Colleen's current lab work and the nutella did the trick. At her next clinic visit Colleen is back to her cheerful little girl self and Grandma gives me a hug. The oils in the nutella coat the taste buds and the second spoonful of nutella helps mask the after-taste. It is times like these that make working as an AIDS Nurse a pleasure. Watching patient's young and old thrive is a whole lot better then having to prepare them for death.

# 1998
# Future Dr. Mike

Rev. Bruce Davidson of the Lutheran AIDS Task force, asked me to do a presentation on making good choices for a Jersey City youth group of boys and girls ages 13-to -17. The presentation is about 45 minutes; I keep it short and on point. When I finish, there's time for a Q&A. I see that they are hungry for the information I give them.

I'm about to leave and a young teenager named Michael Ruzek, stops and asks if he can speak with me privately. He asks, "Mr. Varsalone, you work at Newark Beth Israel, right?"

"Yes".

"Is that the one they call 'the Heart' Hospital of New Jersey? He asks.

"Yes,"

Michael then asks if they have a summer mentorship program. I really don't know the answer to that, so I tell Michael I will let him know. I ask him why he wants to know and he tells me his favorite uncle in Egypt died of a heart attack and he wants to become a cardiologist. I can't believe this young teenager knows exactly what he wants to do in life. I give Michael my card and tell him to call me in a week while I search for an answer.

On the following Monday I request a meeting with the Vice President of Nursing. I ask if we have such a program.

"We do if you would like to start one," she says.

I love a challenge so I go to work on it right away. Michael calls me exactly one week later. I am able to tell him: "Last week we did not have a program, but we have one now. Michael, you will be the first to pioneer it."

The nursing department approves my plan for that summer. Kathy, one of the nurses in the Cardiac Cath. Lab is excited to work with Michael all summer and start making a cardiologist out of him. Michael works in the lab and is able to become certified in CPR. At times, the cardiologists take him into the procedure room and let him watch. Since we both live in Jersey City I pick Michael up and drop him off at his family's home on Vroom Street. By the end of the summer Michael is convinced he wants to go to medical school. Michael and I have many conversations during these trips back and forth and he becomes like a son to me.

He is now Dr. Mike and is working in a major hospital in New Jersey. Even though Michael credits me for that opportunity, I must say any young person who is keen enough to know what path they want to take in life has to get the credit for it. In my younger years I never knew what path I wanted to take in life.

# 1968
# Fear Among the Flowers

It happened back when I was 11years old. It was spring 1968, and I had recently started working at Delea's Flower Shop on West Side Avenue. That's where I met one of my best childhood friends, Pasqual. We went to different schools but were the same age. Pasquale went to Our Lady of Mount Carmel in the Marion section, where many Italians lived. Pasquale was always the tough guy.

Every other 11-year-old either respected him as I did, or feared him. Even at such a young age I emulated Pasquale and

wanted to be just like him, so I lived vicariously through him
when it came to being a tough guy.

I was the kind-hearted type. I'm not really sure why, but
Pasquale really took a liking to me right from the first day we
met at Delea's. He was there before I was, so I just followed his
lead. That was easy because Pasquale was a real leader in everything he did.

I probably had a crush on Pasquale and didn't even realize
it. At the flower shop, we watered the plants, carried deliveries
from the trucks and handled the cash register. Mr. Delea was an
older man maybe in his early 70's and he needed young kids like
us to do the heavy work. He was a nice man and obviously a good
businessman because he could pay us a few bucks and get a lot of
hard work out of us. I made more at the flower shop than I did
working at the bingo hall, but I kept both jobs, because bingo
was always held at night. At a young age, I was rolling in dough.

The flower shop was right across the street from the cemetery. Mr. Delia specialized in funeral arrangements; the kind
on the stands that were shaped like a religious cross or chalice.
Sometimes people would call and ask if he could make a flower arrangement look like one of their dead pets. They would
bring in a photo of their deceased pet, Mr. Delea would do it
up for them in flowers and people would cry when they saw the
arrangement.

Pasquale was learning the flower business. His father was a
florist, but he died at a very young age and I remember Pasquale
saying he could run this shop on his own. In my eyes Pasquale
could do anything he wanted. He was handsome, talented, and
unbearably straight.

I liked working in the flower shop and learning the different types of plants and flowers. Everything is seasonal, so in the

spring we had tulips, daffodils, hyacinths and Easter lilies. I loved the lilacs; they had such a nice smell. In summer, we sold geraniums and azaleas, which people would buy and plant on the gravesites of loved ones.

Mr. Delia had special customers who used to come in almost on a weekly basis and buy their own favorite plants for the graves. Pasquale and I would be sent with the customers to go across the street to the cemetery, dig the hole for the flowers, plant them and water them. We would always get a tip when we did that.

On Sundays, the store was usually closed, but this one Sunday, someone famous must have died - a politician or a very popular person. Mr. Delia had a lot of arrangements and deliveries to make. I lived a half a block from the store, so he called and asked if I would mind the store while he was doing these deliveries.

"Keep the 'CLOSED' sign up and water the plants. I'll be back shortly," he said. "We are closed for business, so do not open the door for anyone."

He left me in the store and I began watering the plants. It was just before Easter so there were lots of tulips and lilies. From the back, I heard a hard knock on the door, so I went to the front and one of the regular customers; Mr. Hickey was at the door. I had just planted flowers on his wife's gravesite the day before. I usually saw him on Saturdays when he would get a plant or some flowers and I would go with him to his wife's grave and I would plant them for him. He was very friendly and always gave me a five-dollar tip, which, was megabucks back then. He was probably a rich, lonely guy.

When he knocked and I came out to the front and saw him, I thought something was wrong with the planting I did for him the previous day and he came to tell me to fix it. But how would he know I was there on a Sunday?

Maybe he was walking by and saw me in there. He knocked on the window and I said, "I can't let you in because we're closed."

And he said, "I just want to look at the Easter lilies for next week."

I said, "Okay," and I let him in.

I locked the door and we went in the back. I was trying to pick out the best Easter lilies I could find for my favorite customer. Mr. Hickey was standing behind me. I turned around and he had his penis out. I was numb for a second and could not even speak. All I could think of was how I wish Pasquale were here.

He asked me if I wanted to stroke him and play with his penis. I didn't know what to say. I kept thinking I don't know why this is happening. But I also thought I definitely don't want to lose that five-dollar a week tip, so I better do what he says.

Mr. Hickey was gentle. At first it was just playful, no rough stuff. I was pretty naive at 11 to think that was all it was. I was just starting to experiment with girls. I never realized until then that guys did anything with other guys.

Just as he was bending me over and about to take me from behind, I saw Lea, the younger sister of my friend Will looking in the window. I looked up and yelled, "THERE'S LEA!" and Mr. Hickey zipped up his pants and made me swear never to tell anyone. I went home that day and never told a soul.

Looking back, I believe deep in my heart that if my friend Pasquale had been there that day, this incident never would have happened.

The next evening after school, my grandmother could see something was wrong with me. My face must have told a story and being only 11, I didn't realize it. Sitting in her rocking chair watching her favorite TV show, "The Beverly Hillbillies," she said,

"Figlio Mio, che cosa fa?" which means "My son, tell me what's wrong?"

How did she know? I guess only a grandmother could know, or a mother. My mother didn't seem to notice a difference. How did Grandma know? I don't understand, but she knew something was not right with me.

"Nothing, nothing's wrong," I lied. And she just hugged me and said, "You know that you can tell me no matter what it is." Of course, I never did. At 11, I might have been thinking, is it better to tell her or is it better to keep this quiet because of the possible consequences of people finding out that this happened to me? What would Mr. Hickey say if someone questioned him about this? Back then, adults would look at you and say, "You're wrong. That didn't happen. Why are you making up these stories?" They'd smack you, too. Back then in the 50s and 60s, adults always took the side of other adults and kids were always wrong, always the liars.

My biggest fear was that if I told someone they would accuse me of making it up. At 11, I didn't know what homosexuality was. It wasn't a word ever used at home. The only bad word I knew in my household was "fag" because that's what my brother used to call me. To my understanding, a fag was a sissy not two boys experiencing a sexual encounter. Knowing now what happened to Uncle Mike I sometimes wonder if they would have thrown that Diagnostic and Statistical Manual at me. After all, it was 1968. I could have ended up like Uncle Mickey.

For years I lived with the pain of what happened and kept it a secret. I swore I would never tell anyone. I was going to take the incident at the flower shop to my grave. I first had to figure out a way to find out if Lea saw anything when she looked through the window. I got the sense that she was looking in but didn't see anything.

My little sister loved the telephone and helped me keep a handle on my social calendar. If the calls were from male friends, I always took those calls so I could brag to them that Jane or Jill or Shelly called me. I wanted to boast to the guys in school just in case anyone had any doubts about whether I was a "fag" or a lady's man. I left everyone with no doubt that I was a straight boy. I guess I was a born actor.

Another change happened after the flower shop incident. I seemed to be unable to even look at men. I had no tolerance for them. I had to be around women all the time, girls at school, older women at the Bingo hall where I worked or with my sisters, especially Sue. Of course, there was Mom and most especially Grandma. I don't think there was anyone in the whole world that knew me better or loved me more than she did.

My life as a pre-teen was going along pretty well until the summer of 1968 when Grandma, at age 88, suffered a mild heart attack. She was not in the hospital for too long and soon went back to visiting Uncle Mickey twice a week like she did every week of her life. Grandma continued to cook and clean and pray to every Saint statue in every room of the house every day. At 88 she was still amazing even after the mild heart attack.

I used to love watching her do her morning rituals. First she would say a thank you prayer to God for giving her another day. After that, she walked around the house and kissed every holy statue – and there were lots of them. She would make her bed, drink a cup of black coffee and then make a soft-boiled egg with toast. The left over toast or stale bread she would use to feed the birds.

Opening the kitchen window in the back of the house she would fling the bread to the garage roof. How could she throw that far, I would think to myself? Occasionally she would wet the bread if it was too hard and then hold her hand out the window. At times a little sparrow would come to the clothesline and slowly and cautiously hop along the rope, then take the bread from Grandma's hand and fly away. I tried to do this and it just never worked for me. The birds would sit on the garage roof as if to say "Well, are you going to throw the bread or not?"

In 1968, we made it through the holidays, but grandma seemed to be getting weaker. I was almost a teenager and I was starting to get worried she would die and then what would I do without the person who loved me the most?

# 1969
## Grandma's Stories

January 20th was a cold winter day. Richard M. Nixon had won the presidential election in November of '68 and it was the day of his inauguration. My grandmother got up early in the morning, made her bed, drank her black coffee, said her prayers and then settled down in the living room to watch her favorite shows, none of which were on because it was all about Nixon.

Grandma was very disappointed that her "stories" (soap operas) were not on.

Grandma sat there all day waiting for one of her favorite shows to come on. Later, she got up, made chicken soup, and baked chicken with roasted potatoes for dinner. We ate dinner together and then went our separate ways. I went to my room for a while. Mom was on the phone, my little sister was home and Sue was out. My brother and dad were at the Bingo hall.

I got up from my bed, went into the living room to sit with Grandma for a while. She was complaining to me in Italian about how she had been forced to watch "this Nixon thing" all day. At about 10 pm, I was sitting next to Grandma, put my arm around her shoulder and assured her that tomorrow all of her favorite shows would come on again. She said in Italian, *afootida* (to hell with it!) threw her arms up in the air as she said it and the next thing I knew Grandma slumped over my shoulder. When I realized she was not moving I called out "Mom something is wrong with Grandma."

My mother ran into the living room, picked up the black dial phone on the end table and dialed 911 for an ambulance. Then I got on the phone to call Alice who lived a few blocks away. She ran over to our house so she could go with mom in the ambulance to the Jersey City Medical Center.

I was in my room crying and praying when my dad and brother got home from Bingo. Dad asked what happened and as I was explaining it to him Alice and mom came back home; Grandma was dead.

For all the pain and loss I endured in my life as an AIDS Nurse, that pain does not compare with the pain of losing my grandma.

# Six

## 1998
## Education, the key to the future...

From the day I started at Newark Beth Israel Medical Center's Family Treatment Center, I came to love the idea that people living with AIDS now have a fighting chance. I am no longer feeling depressed watching everyone around me die. Even though many are still dying I now have the feeling that as a nurse in AIDS Care, I can participate in helping people live with HIV/AIDS. I love the people I work with and the patients most often bring much joy into my life. I am seeing many people thrive. AIDS is now considered a chronic illness and the fight turns toward prevention of HIV. My focus is beginning to change from helping people die with dignity to having those living with HIV teach others by publically telling their stories. Empowering and educating people about this virus are the future.

## 1999
## Tall Man on Campus

Clinics at Newark Beth Israel in the winter are typically slow because many of the patients have no transportation, and since this last week of January is extremely cold, the waiting room is empty.

I'm in the clinic with the Medical Director, and two other nurses, and we are drinking coffee with the receptionists Cathy and Donna while waiting for a new patient.

"He probably won't come," the usually optimistic Cathy says.

I look at the appointment book and notice the patient's address is just a few blocks from where I live. And just as I look up, through the front door walks a very tall, thin man in a Navy Pea coat wearing a blue cap and a red wool scarf. He takes a seat in the waiting room. I pick up my clipboard, walk over and introduce myself.

"Hi, I'm Nurse Dominick, can I ask how tall you are?"

"I'm 6-foot, 7 inches," he says, laughing.

"Okay shorty," I tell him. "Follow me, and let's get started."

We walk to one of the examining rooms and I proceed to do his intake. His name is Robert, and he is one of the nicest people I have ever met.

"Where do I start?" he says, softly. "I am not a very good person, Nurse Dominick. I was married and cheated on my wife with women – and men. My wife and I had a daughter who died. I started doing drugs, drinking too much, and always making the wrong decisions. When my wife found out I was seeing men she left me. I feel this is totally my fault.

"When I found out I had AIDS, I moved to New Jersey to get away from my scary life in New York," he continued. "In Jersey, I don't know many people, but I start to get into the same habits with the people I'm meeting. One day I land in Clara Maas Hospital in Belleville. I had PCP pneumonia and it was so bad, they thought I'd never recover. I made myself a promise that if I did recover I was going to quit all that and turn my life around.

"I was dying in Clara Maas and this little nun comes to see me. I'm not a religious person, but this little nun asks me if I want to pray with her. At first I thought I was dreaming, but she was real, like Mother Theresa. I was so sick, down to 100 pounds. Can you imagine this big body like that? All bones. I knew I was fading and here is this little miracle worker telling me I'm going to be fine. She tells me to pray on my own and fight for my life, and leave the rest to God. My doctor came in and told me they wanted to try a different medication and needed my approval. I thought, what do I have to lose? After a few more weeks in the hospital, I was feeling good enough to go home. The day I was discharged, I wanted to thank the nun for sticking with me, but I couldn't find her."

"When I got to my apartment, there was a padlock on the door, I had been in the hospital so long. A friend of mine let me stay at his place for the night and took me to his social worker the next day. She called the landlord and explained that I was sick and he has no right to lock me out. He let me back in".

"I really want to change my life, so here I am, ready to see the doctor."

My jaw dropped. I was moved by his story and had to compose myself in order to tell him, "You, sir, are a miracle."

Robert sees The Medical Director who prescribes him a new three-drug regimen with Protease Inhibitors and Non-Nucleoside Reverse Transcriptase Inhibitors. Because of the Protease Inhibitors, people are no longer dying from AIDS. Instead, AIDS has become a chronic illness and people are now living with AIDS.

We have pillboxes from the drug companies to hand out to patients, so I give one to Robert and as was my system, I use different colored jelly beans to represent each of his medications. He will be taking over 20 pills a day with this three-drug regimen and that can be very confusing. I give him a slip for his first blood work, and an appointment for the next month.

Before he leaves, I tell him about Project H.E.L.P. Robert would be a wonderful asset to my group I think, and I'm sure we could help him stay clean and sober as long as his will to live stays stronger than the temptation for drugs and alcohol.

"It's in Jersey City and from your demographic information I see that you live really close to me so I can pick you up on Mondays if you would like to join."

Robert calls me the next day and tells me he wants to come to the Project H.E.L.P. meeting. That next Monday, I pick him up, and he becomes a regular every Monday. He especially loves Ms. Florence. He seems to have found a new mom in her.

## Times they are a Changin'

It's a brisk Monday in March and I'm feeling a little sad because it's the last day for Project H.E.L.P. I'm starting Positive Connection in May, which is reassuring, but I also know there's going to be a lot of drama over the new group.

I drive Robert home after the last meeting of Project H.E.L.P., and he says to me: "You know Dominick, you don't always have to be a participant in someone else's drama."

This is how I learn from the group members every time we meet. I may be helpful to them by giving them information, but sometimes I think they help me more.

Our first meeting of Positive Connection is Monday, May 3 at St. John's Episcopal Church in Union City. Father Steven Giovangelo is the priest and he along with his life partner Jerry welcomed us into the parish Italian style. I'm President and co-founder, Florence is Vice President and co-founder, and Bob is Secretary/Treasurer of the new group. At our first meeting, 11 people show up – eight group members and three volunteers. By May 30, we are already putting together the first Positive Connection newsletter that includes an essay on what I've learned so far running the group, my favorite poem "If" by Rudyard Kipling and two articles relating to HIV-prevention.

# 2000
## Silent Angel of Care...

It's been six years since I graduated from Christ Hospital School of Nursing and I decide I want to want to set up a scholarship fund to give something back. I name it the "Silent Angel of Care" as I want it to be anonymous.

I went to see Carol Fasano who was still Director of Nursing and told her about my idea of giving a scholarship every year for a student who displays care and compassion.

She graciously accepted my offer and added, "by the way, we're looking for a part-time skills lab instructor in the evenings; I'd like to offer you the job."

She told me the particulars. I would be instructing the students on the proper techniques for everything from hand washing to basic nursing procedures in nursing care. I would take the skills I learned over the years, in school, and from practical experience, and bring those skills to students just starting out.

I gladly accepted her offer.

A few weeks into it, I asked a student what they were being taught in class about HIV? When she told me what they were teaching, I realized it was the same thing they taught when I was in nursing school. I just couldn't stand by without doing something about it.

I immediately went to Grace Franne, she was the coordinator of the nursing program, and I asked if I could give the AIDS lecture to the senior class. I wrote a curriculum, presented it to her and she loved it. Till this day, the senior class gets a four-hour lecture strictly on AIDS. I start every lecture by saying to the students: "If you have had unprotected sex, even one time, with someone whose HIV status is unknown, then you have exposed yourself to the AIDS virus.

The lecture included medications used in treating patients with HIV/AIDS, opportunistic infections, nursing interventions in all stages of the disease along with prevention, education and empowerment of AIDS patients. I submitted 40 questions to Ms. Franne and she chose several questions for the exam following my lecture.

I also put the 1-800 hotline number on the board. By the end of each lecture, many of the students ask me where the nearest HIV testing site is because they know that somewhere along the line they have unknowingly exposed themselves to the virus and that's how I know what I'm doing is effective. If I could save one life per lecture, it would be a worthy goal.

Every nurse should be asking these types of questions of their patients, especially if their health history warrants it. If I can borrow a phrase from Dr. Carl Kirton, one of my nursing mentors, "Because today, like it or not, every nurse is an AIDS Nurse."

## Patient Advocate

As the saying goes, "One door closes and a new one opens." I still love my job at Newark Beth Israel, my co-workers are great, and the patients are thriving,

It's Thursday, Aug. 10, and Leticia comes in for her clinic appointment. While doing her chart, I notice her viral load has gone from undetectable to 1,200. Although this looks like a huge difference, it's what we call a viral load blip. We're used to seeing numbers of 1 million, even more with some patients. I know right away our Medical Director is going to take her off Combivir, which is a two-drug cocktail in one pill taken twice daily. I also know he will put her on a new three-drug combination that will most likely reduce her viral load to undetectable again and probably raise her T-Cell count high enough to keep her safe from acquiring any of the opportunistic infections. This is the new wave of HIV/AIDS treatment in the new Millennium and everyone is riding it.

It's a regular clinic day, and I take Leticia to an exam room to assess her vital signs and talk to her about her blood work. I tell her that the doctor will probably put her on some new medications because of her increasing viral load. I take out a new pillbox for her and some different colored jellybeans the same way I do for the many others who are being changed from two drugs to three.

Despite her increased viral load that is fairly common, this patient feels great and is ready to see the doc. After her exam, he comes out of the room and gives me her new prescriptions, and asks me to do the medication education. As I re-enter the exam room the patient is sobbing.

"What's wrong?" I ask her, "Why are you crying?"

She then tells me, "I won't do it. I want my Combivir back."

By this time the clinic is backing up with patients and we need the exam room. The Doc starts to huff-and-puff and I think he's ready to blow the door down. I hear him loudly tell other staff members, "He does this to me all the time," insinuating I spend too much time with the patients. Imagine that, a nurse spending extra time with a patient!

I ask Kim, my favorite social worker if we can use her office and we move our conversation there. The patient insists she will not take the new medication, and wants to continue taking the Combivir. I tell her I will try to explain her feelings to the chief in charge, her doctor.

I wait until he finishes with his next patient and I go in to advocate for Leticia.

"Excuse me, Dr.?" I said in a timid voice, knowing from experience what was coming if I try to make a suggestion?

"What do you want now?" he snorts.

"The patient does not want to take her new meds and wants to stay on Combivir," I tell him.

"Well you go tell her that if she doesn't take them to go find a different doctor."

"I will not do that," I say.

"Well then what do you want me to do?"

"I have a suggestion," I tell him. "Is it okay if for just two weeks we keep her on the Combivir and redo her blood work to see if the viral load comes back down to undetectable?"

The next thing I know he slams the chart down, stands up over me and screams so loud that everyone in the clinic and waiting room hear it. "WHAT DO YOU KNOW, YOU'RE JUST A NURSE!"

I'm so angry at him that I think about hitting him; my face is red from the top of my baldhead to the bottom of my neck.

I excuse myself and go into the bathroom down the hall to splash cold water on my face. First I was angry, then humiliated, and even when I calm down I want revenge. This is so uncharacteristic of me.

I go back to Kim's office to talk with the patient. Everyone is looking at me and wondering what's going on. I can still hear the Dr. mumbling, "How dare he?" and "Who does he think he is?" and so on.

I calm down enough to talk to my patient. She says to me, "I'm so sorry Dominick I didn't mean to get you in trouble." I tell her, "Trouble? Girl, this is our boss on a good day."

I devise a plan, but I need Leticia's full cooperation and permission to pull it off. I know after he treated me that way that I plan to leave that job anyway, because there is just no way I am going to be abused by him again.

I ask Leticia if she can keep what I am about to tell her from anyone and she promises. I tell her that legally I have to write in her chart that she is refusing the prescribed treatment. She is fine with that.

I then tell Leticia she should continue taking her Combivir for two weeks without missing a dose. She is perfectly fine with that, too. I give her a slip for her blood work to be done in two weeks, and a new appointment in three weeks so I can check her viral load again. I ask her to take the prescriptions, but not to take them to the pharmacy until after we see her results from the viral load test. Again, she is good with my plan. I let Leticia know that if her viral load comes back to undetectable, she might be able stay on the Combivir, but if it goes up even slightly, she needs to reconsider the three-drug combination that the doctor gave her. She totally agrees.

Two weeks go by and Leticia has the test done, and by the middle of the following week her results are back in and I'm the first to see them. Just as I expected, the viral load is undetectable. She comes in for her follow-up and the doctor takes her chart and shows me the labs that I input into her chart. He gives me a look that seems to say. "See, I was right." He says to Leticia, "I see your new medication is working already."

"Oh no doctor, I never even took those prescriptions to the pharmacy," Leticia says. "I just kept taking the Combivir. I told you I was not going to take all those pills."

He looks my way and I say right in front of the patient, "that's what I tried to tell you three weeks ago." The patient always has the final say about what goes into his or her body.

I know he's livid with me, but I don't care. I wrote my resignation the night of the incident; it's in my pocket.

The next day I come to work and I can't wait for the arrogant doctor to come in. I call the two directors of the clinic, and invite them to see him with me to witness my next move. The doctor is sitting at his desk and the three of us stand in front of him.

The directors have no idea I am about to resign. I look at the doctor and say, "You were right Dr., I am just a nurse. I am just a nurse who cannot work for you. Here is my resignation and my two weeks notice. My resignation is effective Friday, September 15th." You could hear a pin drop. My only regret is that I really like working here, but not under these conditions.

# Right Place, Wrong Time:

It's the weekend and I have some stomach and back pain that won't go away. It finally gets so bad; I have to call an ambulance. They take me to Clara Maas Hospital and the ER attending physician is Dr. Nadir Moaven, who is also the doctor I know from Broadway House. I'm in the ER having a kidney stone attack and he sees me there on a stretcher with an IV solution running through my veins. He asks me if I'm working and I tell him, "not at the moment!"

He laughs and then tells me he needs help with his charts. Apparently his nurse quit and left him in a bind. I tell him I will stop by his office when I'm feeling a little better and we can talk.

I do just that the following week and by the end of August, I start working for Dr. Moaven two days a week. It's very similar to the clinic at Newark Beth Israel except his is a private practice.

# My Journey as an AIDS Nurse

My job is to pre-check vital signs, prepare charts and get all the patients ready to see the doctor. The biggest problem I see is that the waiting time for his patients is deplorable. This is due, in part, because he does not have a nurse setting up the clinic for him before he gets there. I initiate some easier ways of doing things that work with the phlebotomist, and the receptionist. Soon the waiting time is reduced from 90 minutes to 15 minutes, on average.

Things are going well for us and I go from two days a week to full-time for almost a year. I was working days at both offices of Dr. Moaven in Belleville, NJ and in Maplewood, NJ. I was also working evenings as a skills instructor and guest lecturer at Christ Hospital School of Nursing.

On September 11, 2001 I arrive early for work, as usual, but almost none of the patients show up. Everything here on the east coast has gone topsy-turvy. Thousands of people who lived here and in Manhattan and commuted to the World Trade Center are either dead or missing because of terrorist attacks on the World Trade Center twin towers in NYC. I of course, did not know anything until I turned on the television in the waiting area of the Maplewood office.

Knowing Bob works just a few blocks from the towers I call him. I was relieved when he answers but then lost contact with him for the rest of the day. Bob was able to contact his mom in Iowa and she in turn contacted me just to let me know he was still alive. What Bob did not tell his mom I found out only when he returned home about 7PM. He had to walk through the ash and dust on his way to the tugboat that would bring him to Hoboken. He was then washed off with a hose in Hoboken before they would let him come home to Newark. I cannot explain the emotion of this in writing. Bob's clothes were soaking wet but he was

159

still alive, in that moment that was all that mattered to me. In the days to come we, like so many others, mourn those we knew who did not make it that day and we praise God for many others we knew who did make it.

In the weeks after the attack, Dr. Moaven has to let me go. Many of his patients did not come in for appointments and he has to make some cuts. I love working here but he could only pay half of what I was making at Newark Beth Israel Medical Center. I know I am working in the right place but it is the wrong time as it turns out. I know too that Dr. Moaven does not want to let me go but it was what needs to be done for both of us.

Leaving his office with a cardboard box of items from my desk, I think about the years I spent being in the wrong place at the wrong time. I had spent all of those years working on the railroad, unaware of my sexuality or my real life's purpose.

# 1974
## Oil Pans

After high school graduation, my initial dream was to be a United Nations interpreter and I wanted to go to college to study foreign languages, so I applied to McGill University in Montreal, Canada, which offered foreign language degree programs. I could just imagine them laughing at my high school transcript when they saw my "C" average. Of course, in high school, I was more concerned with how popular I was, not how smart.

I didn't get into McGill or any of the other colleges I applied to, so my father said, "Son, you'll have to work on the railroad with me," and I applied for a job at the Penn Central Railroad in Kearny, New Jersey. I was an 18-year-old apprentice railroad man and a good Italian kid following in the footsteps of his father.

# My Journey as an AIDS Nurse

I remember my first day driving to work with my father. We stopped to get buttered rolls and coffee at the corner deli and as we got back in the car, he decided it was time for a heart-to-heart talk with his son.

"Listen, Dominick, I just want you to know that when we're at work, I can't show you no favors."

"I know that, Dad," I said, looking straight ahead at the road, "I don't expect any favors."

"It's not that I don't want to help you out," he said, "it's just that the other guys will bust my chops 'til Kingdom Come if they think I'm doing anything special for you."

"Sure, I understand," I reassured him.

"Now, listen carefully," he whispered, as if he was about to tell me the combination to Fort Knox. "If you need anything, if you have any problem whatsoever, you go to 'Red' the shop foreman. He'll help you. This way it won't look like I'm doing something nice for you. Got it?"

"Sure, Dad. Thanks."

It turned out just like he said. If I had a problem with my shift or had to take a personal day for some reason, I went to Red (Walter E. Kimball, with the red hair), the general foreman. I remember there was a union rule that if you worked more than 15 minutes past your shift, you got paid three hours of overtime at time-and-a-half. It didn't matter if you worked twenty minutes or 2-1/2 hours, if you got your work done, you were paid for three hours. When I had to hand in my time card to my father, he would never pay me the over-time. Even when I worked the full three hours, he wouldn't do it for fear someone would think he was treating me special. He did it for every other guy, but he just couldn't give me those three hours – and that was big money back then – but when Red was in charge of time cards, I would get it.

161

My father would do favors for everyone else, but he wouldn't do them for me. Any favors Red did for me, he rarely did for anyone else. I guess that's why I always felt close to Red and he always felt close to me. I did understand why it had to be that way though.

When I started on the railroad, Red was determined to mold me into the premier railroader. I'm not sure he was convinced that could happen. He knew I had other interests outside the railroad. I wasn't my father. Your typical railroader is usually not into theatre and fashion.

In the early 1970s, freight train repairmen were mostly European immigrants, old laborers with strong backs who weren't afraid of getting their hands dirty. It was rough work. I was a maintenance apprentice making great money watching other people work. That's how you learned on the railroad. You apprenticed with someone experienced. One partner would do all the work and the other would hand over the tools, watch and learn.

If I encountered something I had never seen before, they would be right there to explain it again and again if necessary. That lasted all of six weeks and then the real work began. I think the only real concern I had in those six weeks was how the hell was I going to fill my father's shoes. All of my young life hearing him tell me I would never amount to anything, and here I am with the task of having to live up to his expectations and hearing other maintenance men say things like "you'll go far if you're half as good as your dad."

The job on the railroad was very dirty. I'd have to get up at 5 am to be at work at 6 o'clock, working until 3 pm with a half-hour off for lunch. My workday started in a dirty, greasy locker room. It was horrible. Cold, no heat and there was no thrill watching old men walk around with their asses hanging out. Of course, in my mind, all the old men were dirty old men like Mr. Hickey from my childhood. It was actually frightening at times.

They were pretty free walking around and at the end of the day the old men would shower and get changed, making comments like what they were going to do with their wives or girlfriends when they got home—just to show how macho they were. Just what I needed: a bunch of guys swinging their junk in front of me. I knew even back then that the only reason they all showered after work in those locker rooms was because their wives would not let them back in the house in their dirty clothes. I would change out of my coveralls in the locker room, but I took my showers at home.

The next day, I'd do it all over again – put on my coveralls, and get my assignment from my father who was the billing clerk. He seemed to want to prove some macho point, so he would give me the toughest jobs, everything from greasing wheels to crawling under boxcars on my back to check for cracks under the chassis. Sometimes I'd find the cracks and weld them. As time went on at Penn Central Railroad, I was eventually teaching the new apprentices.

My dad did one great service for me during my time there. Handing out the work assignments, he always placed me with the best teachers, the guys who worked the hardest, like John Olivieri, Willie O'Dell and Walter Reichert.

Shortly before the end of my first year, Penn Central merged with seven other companies to form Consolidated Rail – better known as Conrail. There was a lot of insecurity among the railroad repairmen, especially the older men who worked there for many years, including my dad.

As the merger took place, we were told there would be layoffs and buyouts and most of the old-timers were asked to retire.

My dad, who had over 30 years of service and was about to turn 60, decided to accept the offer. The deal was that anyone who worked thirty years and was 60 years old – or older – could retire with full pay. The men who took the buyout left younger guys with one-two years' experience to teach the new hires. Red was then promoted to Master Mechanic for the entire Northeast Corridor.

Around this time, Lidia my girlfriend was going to the School of Visual Arts in Manhattan where she met a diverse group of artists, many of them handsome gay men. Lidia and I saw each other on a regular basis and were getting along pretty well. We were happy, or at least I thought we were.

# 1975
# How Did He Know?

When several top executives from South Kearny Railway, a privately owned rail system headquartered in Chicago, came to Conrail looking for a field maintenance supervisor, Red recommended me as the best possible choice, and I got the job. Of course, this created animosity among my co-workers because they knew Red was close to my dad and it didn't matter that I was only concerned with inspecting and maintaining the flat cars and that was *not* part of their job. As far as they were concerned, my new job was a 'cake' job that I didn't earn with only two years under my belt. They also didn't like that I would be supervising their work.

Before I took my new position, Lidia and I were engaged. I was 19.

I had been working for a year-and-a-half, saving money like crazy and I was about to give Lidia her engagement ring. It was early November 1975 and I was ushering at St. Bridget's Bingo in Jersey City to make extra money. Every week, Robbie D, a very handsome guy with golden blond hair and his wife, Janet, would come to Bingo and we'd chat between games. It turned out that Robbie was gay; Janet was his close friend – and "beard".

I think I was attracted to him, but I didn't really know at the time. I felt such a connection with both Janet and Robbie that I decided they would be the first people to see Lidia's engagement ring. They complimented my taste and told me Lidia will love it, and then later Robbie took me aside.

"Let's take a ride after Bingo and have a drink to celebrate," he said.

I felt very comfortable with him, and said yes.

We had a connection of some kind, but I did not understand it fully. Did I know he was gay? No, but I do know our attraction to each other made me feel really good. After Bingo, he and I got in his van and drove to Greenwich Village.

"Don't get married. Don't get engaged. Don't give your girl-friend a ring," he said, as we were driving through the Holland Tunnel to Lower Manhattan.

"What? Why?"

"You're too young to get married."

"Why are you telling me this?"

Then he said, "Did you know I was gay?"

"No," I said. "I thought you and Janet were married."

"No, we're just very good friends," he said, pausing for what seemed like forever.

"Do you know that you're gay?" he said to me.

"What? Uh…no." I stammered. "I'm not gay. No way. I've never been with a man or even thought about a man."

I lied.

"You never had sex with a man?"

"No."

"Do you want to have sex with me?"

"No."

"Would you allow me to have oral sex with you?"

"What? Are you crazy?"

"I don't want to do this just to have sex with you or to lead you on," he said. "I just know you are gay. Why don't we do a sort of test?"

"A test? Look Robbie, I like you, but I really don't think I would like oral sex from a guy."

"Has Lidia ever done that for you?"

"Yes!"

"Okay, can you at least close your eyes and pretend it's her mouth?"

"Well I guess I could let you try," I said.

And he did.

I was petrified and my heart was pounding so hard. Was it fear of getting found out or fear that I would like it?

"Did you like that?" he asked.

"Yes I did," I told him. "I liked it a lot. It was amazing, not like anything I ever felt."

"Would you like to try it with me?" he asked.

"Uh…no."

"Okay," he said. "I won't force you because, I'm not doing this for me. I'm trying to save you from a big mistake. I was married when I was really young and I regret that I ruined her life and mine."

We went to a gay bar called Badlands. By now it was 2 am and I admit I was enjoying my time with him. At The Badlands I was also intrigued with all the good-looking guys in the bar. Everyone was kissing or snuggling up with each other and it was making me feel like something might be missing in my life. I heard all the names guys were called for being gay and I had been called those names, too, but I had no idea this is what it was all about. I was so naïve, so vulnerable, and yes very horny from all the excitement.

Back in the van for the second time, Robbie again asked if I wanted to try anything with him. I was too nervous. We did stay there for two more hours and talked, laughed, we even cried.

Robbie and I bonded.

When he pulled up in front of my house to drop me off, it was almost morning and I was hoping he and I would get together again, but it wasn't in the cards.

Robbie's last words to me were "I really like you, and I know you are gay. Someday you will know, too, and you will remember this night and thank me for it."

He was right, as I had found out a few years later, but still Lidia and I were married.

# 1977
# I do?

On May 7, I became a married man. It was official: I was straight. It was six days before my 21th birthday and one week after starting my new job at South Kearny Rail. I am certain if I were not engaged to get married, I would not have been hired there, marriage was almost like a prerequisite. Our married life was what I thought of as normal. Lidia and I saved for a house (someday) like everyone else, and we celebrated every little thing that happened in our lives. We did everything together for almost two years. So many people asked me if I loved my wife, and the answer is yes! But you know the old saying, "If you can't love yourself, you cannot really love someone else." The problem was I did not know at that time how to love myself. Once my true self emerged, the shit hit the fan.

# 1979
## I don't

Lidia and I were involved in Jersey City's local theater scene. She was a wonderful artist and designed scenery. I built the scenery and hung lights (I'm pretty good at swinging a hammer). We were working behind the scenes during the shows, too, and sometimes I got cast. There was a guy on the stage crew with me, Charlie; I didn't know he was gay. He was living with a woman, so I thought he was straight and they were sleeping together. A young guy and a young girl living together, they're probably doing it, right? Then the woman Charlie was living with moved out and my wife started hitting on him.

I found out on Valentine's Day that she anonymously sent Charlie a bouquet of flowers and cut out the words "Happy Valentine's Day" and "Anonymous" from a magazine, knowing that her beautiful and distinctive handwriting would be easily found out. I was home cooking a Valentine's Day dinner – steaks cut in the shape of a heart – when my doorbell rings and Charlie is standing there with a bouquet in his hands.

"Can I talk to you?" he asks.

"Sure," I tell him, "Come on in." He steps inside looking very nervous and I have no idea where this is leading.

"I have to tell you something," he begins. "I hope I'm wrong, but I think your wife is coming on to me."

A little stunned by his remark, I put on my best poker face and say, "Really, what makes you think that?"

"She stops at my job at Blimpie Base," he says. He was managing the Blimpie Base in Journal Square at the time. "She stops in every morning and gets her coffee and she's kind of flirty."

"She's flirty. That's okay. She's being friendly," I reply.

Then he holds out the bouquet as evidence. "Today, these flowers arrived. It's creatively done. I just think she sent these to me."

There was the envelope with the handmade card inside that said "Happy Valentine's Day." Inside in the same kind of cutout words from magazines it read, "I would like to put my mouth around your Blimpie." Did Lidia really send him this? I couldn't believe what I was seeing and hearing, but something inside me told me she did.

I told Charlie, "If you really think this is true, I will use the bouquet as a centerpiece for our Valentine's dinner and see her reaction."

I told him I was okay with this no matter what happened, and that we would remain friends. Charlie left, still looking very nervous and I put the Valentine note attached to the flowers on the table and waited for Lidia to come home.

When she came home from work, she walked into the kitchen, saw the flowers on the table and gasped.

"So you did send these to Charlie?" I asked.

She admitted it and started to cry.

"You know I'm okay with it. I'm not going to fly off the handle. I would just like the respect that if I'm not satisfying your needs, you tell me," I said. "We have to communicate these things."

We sat down to our heart-shaped Valentine's dinner and talked about our now, crumbling marriage. Lidia said she was a nymphomaniac and always wanted more sex than any one man could give her.

"It's not all bad," I told her. I loved her enough to let her experience what she needed to experience, sexually or otherwise, and if that had to be with another person, then we would have to work something out.

Still, in the back of my mind, I was thinking of something my sister said to me not long after we were married "You better put a leash on your wife."

When I asked her what she meant, she said, "I think she's cheating on you with someone at work." I had no idea Lidia was fooling around with some guy who my sister knew. It ended up, she was seeing this guy John at the same time she was hitting on Charlie.

How did I get myself into this mess? I am sure it was partly my fault, because it takes two to mangle a relationship. I should have seen the red flags, like the time we were dating in high school and she drew me that caricature of a girl crying with the caption underneath, "If you don't love me, con me." It didn't turn me off. Instead, I was intrigued and something inside me said I should not let her down.

During the whole time we were dating, she would always make references to her weight and say, "You'll never love me enough to marry me," or "I'll never find anyone as good as you." These conversations always made me feel that if I dumped her it would send her self-esteem spiraling downward.

I realized from all this that one of the reasons I wanted to get married so bad was that I wanted to prove to my father I could be a hardworking man like him and make him proud of me. I was so much like my dad in so many ways.

I've always been a communicator and I believe there's a solution to every problem, so I told Charlie he was right. It was Lidia who sent the Valentine flowers and I invited him over for dinner to discuss it. Lidia admitted to having a crush on Charlie and said she wanted to experience making love with him. She also told me Charlie was responding to her sexual advances that I really did not believe. We talked and I said to him, "If you want to be with my wife, I'm okay with it. Have a good time. I'm totally okay with it."

He looked at me square in the eye and said, "I don't want her. I'm gay. If I'm going to be with anybody it's going to be you."

I was really confused and flattered at the same time. I was never one to give in to rumor. It was a dose of reality and it sent me back to what my friend Robbie told me that night in his van.

Did Charlie also see something in me that I refused to see?

A few years later I ran into Robbie at a gay bar in Manhattan, he was the bartender. We recognized each other right away. That's when I heard what I should have heard back in 1975, the big "I told you so." I still can't understand how everyone knew but me.

# Another Openin', Another Show

So here I am still married, but life was very different in my head. From February to May, Lidia and I tried to come to some kind of agreement. Meanwhile, she had a very demanding sexual appetite that I don't know if any straight man could handle, let alone a gay man trying to be straight. I had to think of a lot of hot men to pull that off, and during sex, I fantasized about male celebrities like Burt Reynolds and Erik Estrada.

I was not interested in acting out my gay fantasies because I was afraid to explore my interests in men any further than in my thoughts. So, while we were trying to work things out, I just couldn't have sex with her, and she was devastated. Now she really had to find sexual experiences elsewhere.

Living with Lidia and sleeping on the couch, I decided to see a therapist. At the time, Charlie was no longer living with Melanie, and to make life more complicated, the three of us were involved in the show, *Dames at Sea.* I was playing Lucky, Lidia was the set designer and Charlie was the stage manager.

And all these feelings started to snowball. In the meantime, Lidia had become bitter for being found out and was making things difficult for Charlie and me. She would see us together and accuse me of sleeping with him. I assure you while we did spend more and more time together, I was still not convinced I was gay and was certainly not ready to come out if I was. I was also not sleeping with Charlie yet.

During rehearsals for *Dames at Sea,* I started having sexual feelings for him. I was frustrated; trying to understand what was going on. I talked to a friend of mine, Bob O, whom I knew was gay. He recommended me to a therapist in New York City, who also did couples' counseling. Lidia didn't want to go, so I went on my own.

I needed to understand what to do about the mess I was in. I went to see her and she helped me realize I was suppressing my homosexuality and my disgust for men, including my own brother and father. This was largely due to keeping in (for all these years) what happened at the flower shop.

I wanted the happy marriage, the house with the picket fence and I wanted children. But Lidia didn't want kids, which in a sense, diminished my whole purpose for being married and made me think, if I'm not going to have a family what am I doing in this marriage? She even got a diaphragm without telling me. I found the blue case and didn't know what it was. I opened it up but there was nothing in it because the diaphragm was in her. Why did she want a diaphragm? Was it because she didn't want to get pregnant at all or she didn't want another guy to get her pregnant? What if she did get pregnant and I think it's my child and the child comes out looking like Carrot Top? Then what do I do?

While Lidia and I were trying to sort things out, I was still sleeping on the couch. We were not really talking, but not hating each other, either. I imagine it was very frustrating for her. She knew she had to be careful about her adultery, so she probably wasn't getting any, which would be extremely frustrating for her.

It's Sunday, May 13, the closing night of *Dames at Sea* and my birthday. I'm on the couch asleep, nude (I never slept with clothes on). It's the middle of the night and I wake up with Lidia grabbing at my genitals with one hand and a knife in the other.

"I want to have sex with you right now or else," she snarls.

"Okay, okay, put the knife down, go into the bedroom and we'll have sex." I tell her. Then, I get up off the couch and slapped her. I didn't know what else to do. I knew I was not going to have sex with her especially under those circumstances. So, I put on some clothes and left her there, lying on the floor crying.

I went over to Charlie's apartment next door. It was three in the morning. After a minute of knocking quietly so not to wake up everyone in the apartment, he opened his door.

"What's up?" he said.

"Lidia just tried to castrate me!" I'm trembling, very upset. A short time after I got inside and caught my breath, Lidia's pounding can be heard on Charlie's door. She's screaming so all the neighbors can hear her.

"Get out of there you faggot!"

Charlie went outside to talk to her, "I'm not letting you into my apartment."

"He's in there, isn't he? And you two have been fucking this whole time. That's why he won't go near me!"

"No, Dominick and I are not having sex. In fact, he just told me what happened, what you tried to do to him, so consider me a witness."

"I'm calling the cops!" she screams. "Look at this mark on my face."

"Go ahead, call the cops. You're lucky he didn't kill you after what you did to him. And if the cops come, I'm going to tell them it's your fault. I have the proof."

That's because when I left my apartment, I took the knife with me.

The next day, Lidia filed a domestic violence complaint with the police. There was going to be trouble. Up until this time neither of us had told anyone we were having problems in our marriage. I did not tell my family anything up until this point, but that was the end of Lidia's silence.

I am sure she told her family what had transpired the night of my 23$^{rd}$ birthday. The next day, May 14, I found an apartment on Kennedy Boulevard in Jersey City. I had enough money for the security and the first month's rent. Later in the week I saw that all the bank accounts were frozen, obviously Lidia had gone to a lawyer. All I had to my name was a pillow and a blanket.

That afternoon, I made sure our blue Datsun B-210 was gone and I went in and took my clothes and left a note. "I'm gone. I don't want anything in the apartment, just my clothes."

After I cooled down a little bit, I realized I did not take my Grandmother's beautiful antique cedar hope chest, which is all I wanted. I did not think about it at that time because I simply wanted out of the relationship at that point. I was frightened; not knowing what Lidia would do next. Of course her next move was to change the locks. Except for the hope chest everything else was hers to keep.

Charlie was the only person who knew where I was living. No one knew, not even my family. Lidia called my parents and sisters, and just told them I had moved out but did not give a reason. I know she was trying to play it like I just decided to end the marriage and that she had no clue why. In the weeks to come Charlie had given me copies of all the love letters she had written to him and I still have them. These letters would make a sailor blush.

When we first started having trouble in our marriage, Lidia and I had decided not to tell our families we were having these problems. I wouldn't talk about her love notes to Charlie and she promised not to tell anyone I was sleeping on the couch. After the knife incident, all bets were off. I wanted her out of my life for good. I relished the opportunity to figure out what my life was all about including these feelings I was having for Charlie and other men.

On Thanksgiving Day 1979 with my entire family around the dinner table Lidia shows up uninvited. Walking through the unlocked front door, she has decided to out me to my family.

"The reason why Dominick and I are no longer together anymore is because your son is a faggot," she blurted out to my entire family.

Before she walked out my father had to have his say. "If that is true than what good is he to you?" he retorted. "Now get out!"

Lidia left, slamming the door behind her. Without skipping a beat my father looked at me and said, "Pass the gravy."

Shocked by his response to Lidia the whole family just went back to eating dinner. You could have knocked me over with a feather.

# 1990
# Derailed

The transition from railroad worker to AIDS Nurse began when my boss called me saying that if I wanted to keep my job, I would have to relocate to Baltimore. When I explained to him that I had just bought my first house, he said the company would allow me to sell the house and they would pay for the move and everything, but they gave me an ultimatum: move or lose my job.

Bob was still in school at NYU and was not going to graduate with his Masters Degree until May 1992 so there was no way I was going to leave Jersey City for Baltimore. I tried to convince my boss and everyone else I could handle the job from New Jersey without having to move, but they would not agree to that.

So, on October 16, I was asked to meet with the South Kearny Railway lawyers who served me papers and fired me from my job. They had planned to give me a package deal of a week's pay for every year I worked for the company. I also had to give them the keys to the company van.

Speaking with my friend Teresa who was in law school at the time and doing her internship at one of the largest law firms in New Jersey, she told me that I had a lawsuit if I wanted to fight this. Of course, railroading was all I knew and I really didn't want to fight. I wanted to keep my job even as bad as they were making it for me. But I felt that the reason why they were doing this had nothing to do with my job performance and had only to do with the fact that they found out I was gay.

My friend Teresa had suggested a lawyer she had worked with while she was in school who specialized in discrimination suits, a paraplegic gentleman who got around in a wheelchair. Bob and

I met with him in his Chatham office. He was older and seemed really smart and experienced and good at what he did.

He took us into his office and started to ask what he said were going to be very personal questions. He said all you need to tell me is the truth. When I explained the story and told him why I felt South Kearny Railway was discriminating against me based on my being homosexual, he said we had a good case, and was confident he could win it for us.

He said that if it went to full trial by jury, we could build this case to be worth $250,000, or more. He went on to say that we would have to pay him about half of that for his services and that the case could last as many as 10 or 15 years. He asked us if we were sure we wanted to endure the mud we would be dragged through and to have this as part of our lives for many years to come. His insight into these situations helped us make the decision that we would only move forward for the settlement I was offered.

Based on what he said, we decided that we would not allow South Kearny Railway to drag me through the mud. We took the settlement plus accrued vacation, and sick time. They would also have to extend Cobra payments for healthcare up until the time I found employment and if they didn't accept this, we would have to file a suit based on discrimination.

We weren't sure which way South Kearny Railway would go with this, but on the day we met to try and settle this, it was held in a Morris County law office with the South Kearny Railway's lawyer, our lawyer, a judge, Bob and me.

The building was not wheelchair accessible and Bob and I had to carry our lawyer in his wheelchair up the steps in order for him to get into the building. It was an easy task and we thought nothing of it, but to my surprise as our lawyer wheeled himself through the hallway to that conference room, this was the first thing out of his mouth.

"Your Honor, with all due respect, we are here today to fight a suit based on discrimination. And I must tell you, if they don't get a ramp for handicapped people for this office, I will come back and file a suit of my own. Now let's begin."

Our lawyer proceeded to tell the Judge why he thought South Kearny Railway was trying to force me out of my job because I was gay. You could see the South Kearny Railway lawyer's face turning different shades of red as our lawyer spoke. I couldn't believe it then and, sometimes, I still can't believe it. What I thought would be an all-day meeting turned out to be a settlement agreed upon in less than an hour. The money that I received went for three things: pay our lawyer, who was worth way more than we gave him; buy a car because I would no longer be able to drive the company van; and put myself through school, although at that time I had no idea it would be nursing school. We did not come out of this with a fortune but I was so glad it was over. Getting fired from my job for being gay was actually the best change of direction my life ever took.

# More Scenes from My Scrapbook

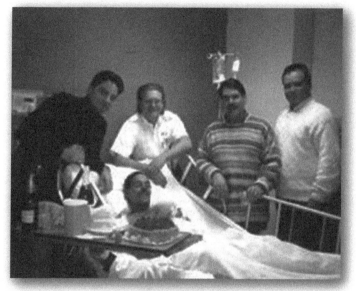

*Jorge's Brother's Birthday*

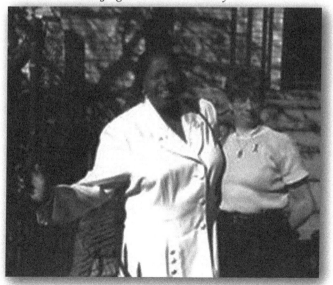

Florence and RoRo

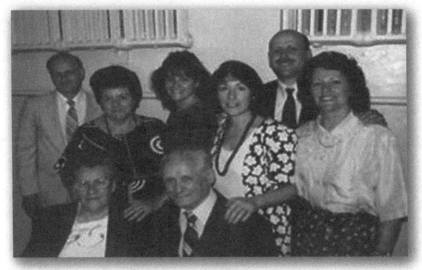

My family

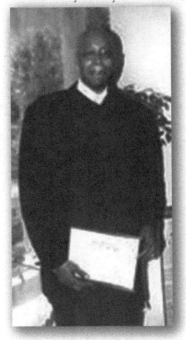

Robert W.

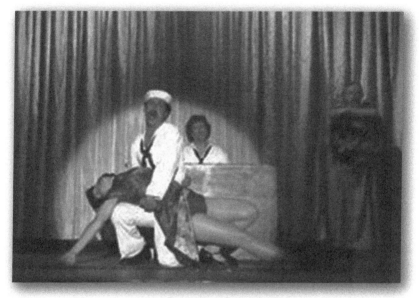

Dames at Sea

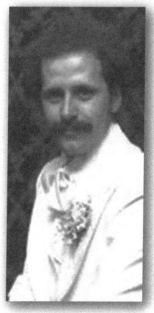

My Wedding Day

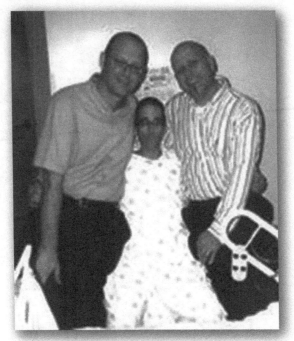

A friends last days

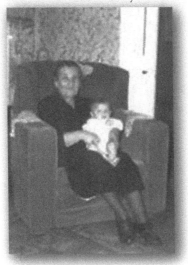

Grandma & little Me

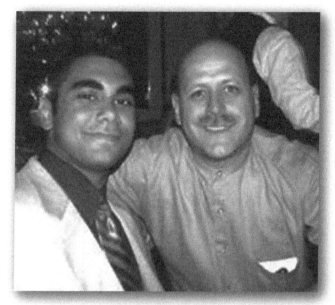

Dr. Mike and Me

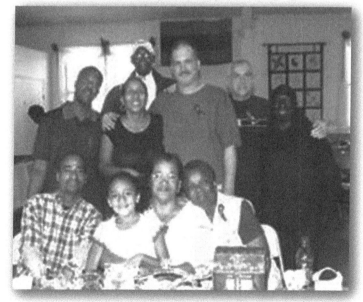

The old Clifton group & volunteers

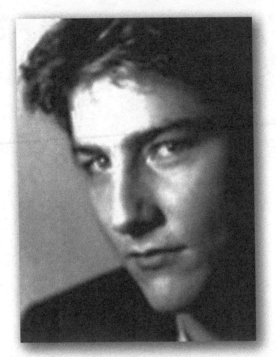

David G.

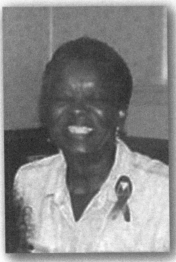

Lovely Lady

# Seven

## 2003
## Do Not Enter

It's Monday, 8:30 am and I arrive at the North Jersey Community Research Initiative (NJCRI) to start my new job as a research nurse. I took the job at NJCRI because of the opportunity to work with Dr. George Perez who I trained under when I first became an AIDS Nurse at Broadway House.

I feel a little nervous to be working at NJCRI because I have no experience in research nursing. At school, they didn't delve into research too deeply, so I will learn as I go along. At least I know Dr. Perez is glad I joined the team. For many years, Dr. Perez has held a 5:30 am AIDS clinic at NJCRI and St. Michael's Medical Center in Newark. He does this for his patients who are commuting to New York City and need to be to work earlier.

Dr. Perez used to handle these clinics by himself, without a nurse, and when Nurse Karen and I volunteered to come in and help him, he was elated. Dr. Perez is an incredible physician who cares about his patients, and treats his nurses with respect and gratitude.

"Thank you nurses," he'll say. "Is there anything else you need me to do before I head upstairs to the hospital?" And then he finishes with, "Okay, then, thank you all for your hard work today."

Dr. Perez, What a class act.

My job at NJCRI is to help carry out clinical research for pharmaceutical trials. There are many different types of clinical trials like Vax-Gen which is testing for a vaccine, SMART which is the Strategic Management of Anti-Retroviral Therapy Study, and finally all of the new combination pill trials being looked at in this time period. A load of new research that is critical for the survival of millions of people in the world who are living with HIV/AIDS. I absolutely loved being a tiny spec in this arena.

This morning, I am working on a brand new study for a new injectable Entry (Fusion) Inhibitor trial called T-20 305, a drug by Roche and Trimeris pharmaceutical companies. The third phase of the study is underway.

I begin with the T-20-305 clinical trial. Each clinical trial nurse was initially given only three patients for this trial. I already have six very sick patients who want to go on this clinical trial and I just do not want to choose only three. I had made an appeal to the head of the study team and as it turned out another clinical trial nurse in my area was not participating in this trial and the powers that be, gave me the three extra patients I requested. The last trial participant I randomized into the study was a man named Trevor who arrives for his first session for self-injection training of this new medication. I greet Trevor in the exam room. We set up all the supplies and we're about ready to start when Trevor starts sweating profusely and looks like he's about to pass out.

Close to tears, he tells me he needs a moment. I bring him a glass of water and he says, "Dominick, I appreciate everything you are doing for me, but I am deathly afraid of injecting myself with a needle. I don't think I can do it, I can't, I just can't!"

Trevor is in end stage, and he has to do this or he will die, so at first I don't know what to say. Then I pick up a syringe, fill it with saline and ask him to watch me inject myself. I tell Trevor I have never injected myself before and, quite frankly, I'm scared, too. We both laugh at how wimpy two grown men can be. I close my eyes, take a deep breath, wipe an area of my left abdomen with an alcohol swab and stick the needle under my skin, as I would have if I were doing a sub-Q injection of a patient.

I look at him and say, "It was really easy and it didn't hurt so now it's your turn." Trevor follows my lead perfectly.

"Wow," he says, "that was way easier than I thought."

I give Trevor his kit and call him every day until his next visit and eventually it becomes so easy for him that he begins to help me help others. Together, we start a focus group for patients afraid of self-injection called *Do Not Enter,* and we hold it at Broadway House in the conference room on Wednesdays. Trevor and I facilitate the group with nurse Karen.

All the physicians in the Newark area who are treating people with HIV/AIDS are contacted. If they are putting their patients on Fuzeon, we tell them to send them to Broadway House to practice self-injection. Every week, a different group stops by. Records are kept as an independent study to measure the program's success.

# 2004
# Out of the Darkness, Into the Light

It's January 4, the first Sunday of the new year, and I'm scheduled to be Cross Bearer on the altar at church, and my job is to take attendance. Halfway through the service, I notice a young man sitting way in the back, in the corner of the last row with his head down. He seems to be crying.

After the service, we do the Sign of Peace, where we greet the person next to us and wish them God's blessing for the coming week. While everyone walks out of the church; this young man sits there.

The minister says to me, "Can you go over and ask what's wrong?

I walk over and ask him, "May I sit down?"

"Yes," he says.

I tell him my name and let him know I'm an altar assistant and I noticed he seems to be upset about something, and would he like to talk about it?

"My name is Carsten, I'm addicted to drugs and I have AIDS and I don't know what to do," he says.

"Okay, let me tell you right up front that it is safe to talk to me," I tell him. "You can tell me anything and no one has to know but you, God, and me. I give you my promise. I also want you to know I'm an AIDS Nurse. Would you like to talk privately?"

"Yes," he says.

We head downstairs to one of the church offices.

I immediately call Bob and tell him I can't come home right away, that there's an AIDS emergency at church. He says, okay, and we agree to catch up when I get home later. That's what's great about Bob. He understands. He knows I have to be where I have to be when I have to be there.

Carsten and I talk. He tells me he has been living with his two sisters, and that he was raised Catholic but rarely ever went to church.

"I had a life once," he tells me. "A really good life, but I got messed up with the wrong people. My sisters will not allow me back in their house because when I need money for drugs, I steal from them – and they've had it with me. My whole family has had it with me. I would go back to my father's house, but if I'm high, he'll call the cops and have me put me in jail."

"Have you been to a drug rehab?"

"No," he says.

"Are you being treated for HIV?"

"Yes," he says. I see a doctor in Paterson, NJ. I know his physician and I ask if it's okay for me to advocate for him, if necessary. He agrees.

I ask if he has ever been to a support group? He says "Once, but it wasn't for me."

I can see Carsten feels comfortable talking with me so I invite him to Positive Connection, which is meeting the next day. It's the first group of the New Year and we always talk about our resolutions.

Carsten tells me that he felt God was pointing him in the direction of the church that morning. "God brought me to the right church today," he says. Then he thanks me, and says, "I will definitely see you tomorrow."

I ask Carsten if he has somewhere to stay tonight and he does, a friend who he says is "safe" and won't tempt him to do drugs.

The next evening, Carsten shows up at Positive Connection and the group welcomes him. He shares his story and at the end, he says he will return the following week.

Carsten also attended a church celebration the next day, Robert and Roro speak about Positive Connection to an audience of nearly 100 people, many of them priests from other churches.

Later that week I receive a call from Carsten telling me he's not going to make it to Positive Connection on Monday. He's not feeling well, he says, and he promises to be at the next meeting.

After Carsten misses a second meeting in a row, I think for sure he's never going to return, but I'm wrong. I should not judge him that way. I know from experience that when a person comes to group for the first time and misses the next week, it's usually because they didn't feel comfortable. That's fine. I know group isn't for everyone.

Carsten comes to the third meeting of the year and tells us he was at the doctor's office and his doctor told him she found K.S. in his femoral lymph nodes when she did a biopsy back in November. He is devastated, and so are we.

Everyone in our group loves Carsten. He's nice, personable, and a decent, good-looking guy. He comes to group faithfully. Unfortunately, just as he's getting used to a drug free time in his life, K.S. is kicking his butt. New medications have him vomiting all the time, and fluid is beginning to build in his ankles. His sisters are worried and think he should be in a nursing home or hospital because they both work and don't know how to care for his medical needs.

## The Devil Made Me Do It

Bob and I decide to take Carsten in and move him into our guest room. He has a TV, and plenty of food, and when I'm home from work he has someone to care for him. Carsten has good days and bad days, but we do the best we can, one day at a time. I know with the K.S. and the swelling of his legs that it won't be long before Carsten will need to be in Broadway House, so I start making calls.

Bob and I have tickets to a New Jersey Devil's hockey game on Feb. 27 that were purchased before we knew Bob would be in Kansas City that day for work. I ask him if he feels strong enough to go to the game with me and he says, "I've never been to a hockey game before."

So we go to the Continental Arena in East Rutherford to see Carsten's first hockey game. We talk a lot; mostly about his addiction and recovery.

Carsten tells me that when he gets a phone call from one of his sisters and does not answer the phone right away, they go into a panic. And sure enough, we're walking into the house after parking the car and his sister calls on his cell phone, screaming, "You're high again, aren't you? You're with that guy Dominick and you're probably getting high with him right now!!"

Overhearing her, I tell Carsten "give me the phone."

"First of all calm down, "I say to her, sternly. "Your brother is fine. I took him to a hockey game. And by the way, I don't do drugs. Your brother is in recovery and he's not doing drugs while he's with me. You need to get over this."

She says, "How come when I call him, he doesn't call me back?"

"I know it must have been rough for you," I tell her, "but as long as he's with me, you don't have to worry. It's important that you trust him, now. Let him handle this."

She hangs up somewhat reassured. I get it. She doesn't know me well and thinks maybe I'm a drug addict, too. She met me only once; I run a support group, big deal.

The next day, He and I go to his sisters' house and I explain exactly what's going on. Everyone in Carsten's family is now good with the fact that he lives with Bob and me, and I think they're relieved as well.

## Tying the Knot Twice

Edgar and his partner have a commitment ceremony at St. John's Church on July 27 with Interim Pastor, the Most Rev. William

Coats, a great friend of Positive Connection, officiating. Positive Connection holds the reception at a local Italian restaurant; Roro made all the arrangements. Edgar's sister Juanita is there to witness the ceremony; her tears reveal how happy she is for her gay brother and new brother-in-law. Everyone is so happy for Edgar, the young man who was given two weeks to live during my early years at Broadway House. Edgar (Baby Boy), the miracle child, is alive and well and hopeful about the future. Every AIDS story should have a "new beginning" like Edgar's.

Another exciting day for Positive Connection is the civil union of Robert and Tanji on February 15 of the following year. Bob and I have the honor of being the witnesses in the ceremony held in the church under God's watchful eye.

Robert has been with Positive Connection for six years and he met Tanji at a function for the Hyacinth Foundation. Tanji was sitting with Anthony Salandra, an AIDS advocate for many years, and Robert and I were sitting at the next table. I excused myself to speak with Anthony and introduced myself to Tanji. I had noticed he was looking at Robert all day and Robert was telling me he wanted to meet Tanji. I suggested to Tanji that he should talk to Robert, and they hit it off immediately. It was a match made in heaven.

Robert and Tanji have been together about five years before their civil union took place. After the ceremony, everyone goes back to Robert and Tanji's apartment where there is plenty of food and lots of dancing. It was a very happy day.

A month later, talk of the most recent Positive Connection wedding is still fresh in our hearts and minds when I receive a call from Robert saying that Tanji is in the hospital and that I should get there as soon as possible. I cannot remember where I am or what I am doing but I drive to University Hospital right away because Robert is too upset to go into detail on the phone.

When I arrive, Tanji is on life support with a sub-dural hematoma he sustained from a fall in the bathtub. He is kept on life support until all of his family can get there to help Robert decide what to do.

I know it is going to be a long weekend of stressful decisions that Robert and the family will have to make and I want to be there for them. I cancel Monday's group not knowing how long it will be before Tanji is out of the coma or taken off life support.

Tanji died the following Monday. He was 45. I know he would want us to say he lived a full life, but he only lived to be 45? How could that be a full life? Tanji became HIV-positive when he was 24. He lived with the virus for 21 years.

Positive Connection meets the following Monday, March 15, which would have been Robert and Tanji's one-month anniversary. It is more of a bereavement group that night. Only 12 people show up. That's because sometimes people can't accept or cope with this type of tragedy. Robert told me he would not be there, but he wants me to provide some gentle healing to the group members that attend.

On the following Monday, Robert is back at Positive Connection and asks every member not to mourn Tanji but to celebrate him. Robert is an exceptional human being of tremendous strength.

## Over the Rainbow

While Carsten stays with Bob and I, he seems to be getting worse. His vomiting has become excessive and his legs are hurting and swelling up. Not acutely ill, Carsten can't be admitted to a hospital or Broadway House because admission there has to be from a hospital only. I call Dr. Perez and ask his advice. He says, "Take Carsten to St. Michael's Emergency Room and have him admitted under my care."

Dr. Perez communicated with Carsten's doctor and they both decided Broadway House would be best, so I call my friend Maggie, the nurse practitioner at Broadway House. I've known Maggie since high school French class with Mr. McGhee.

"What can I do to get him in there?" I ask. "He's dying and needs to be watched 24/7."

Maggie expedites the paper work and we get Carsten in. The whole time he was in St. Michael's he was getting bigger and bigger, from the feet up just like Jorge.

Carsten was a professional tennis player and had a beautiful athletic body. He was very handsome, and it is so difficult to see him deteriorate this way.

Carsten is now settled in at Broadway House receiving palliative care, and his family is there around the clock. We were all there on what would be Carsten's last birthday. I spend much of my time helping his family understand and cope and at the same time, after the loss of Tanji, I'm in need of some rest. I'm glad Carsten is at Broadway House on 2 East because I know Nurse Peggy will watch him closely and let me know when I need to get there.

A few days go by and on May 10 Carsten, now on his deathbed, starts to reach for the sky. I am with him and say, "Are you seeing the white light? Go to the white light. Your family and friends are there."

He says, "I don't see the white light, but I do see a pot of gold at the end of the rainbow." Then he squeezes my hand, stops speaking, closes his eyes, and is pronounced dead a short time later.

I have to design my poster for the upcoming AIDS Conference in Bangkok, Thailand. I take my inspiration from Carsten and put the silhouette of a face in profile and a rainbow going from the head to a pot of gold and the word, "Fuzeon" which is one of the medications Carsten was taking.

At the AIDS conference, I explained the poster's meaning. Carsten's death had an impact. His death, the deaths of all of my friends, and all the other patients I know who died from AIDS, they all made an impact on the disease that took their lives. They were people of all colors, all religions, each had his/her own life and personality. Most important, they were of the same family, "The Human Family."

On June 7, Positive Connection holds a Memorial Tribute to Carsten. The very next day I attend the annual fundraiser for the American Foundation for AIDS Research (AMFAR). While there I have the privilege of meeting Larry Kramer, Kenneth Cole and my favorite actress Meryl Streep. It was held at Gotham Hall in Manhattan on 36th Street. I credit Larry Kramer, Liz Taylor and Elton John along with many other people from AMFAR for saving the lives of thousands of people by standing up to make a difference in the world of HIV/AIDS.

The following day, I receive a letter from the International AIDS Society stating, 'Congratulations. Your poster has been accepted for display at the International AIDS Conference in Bangkok, Thailand.' The life of every nurse is like a roller coaster ride, one day your patient dies, or you get that sinking feeling when a friend calls to say they have just been diagnosed. The next day your hard work takes you to a place where you can learn something new and teach what you learned to people all over the world and try to make a difference. Nurses should be honored all year long not just for one week in May.

## Access for All

Conferences like the International AIDS Conference in Bangkok, Thailand show the small changes and breakthroughs in HIV/

AIDS, the little miracles that happen each and every day all over the world. Organizations represented at the conference have ideas on how to improve the lives of people living with HIV/ AIDS, but not one has a cure. There are many breakthroughs announced at the conference, but no miracles.

I'm proud of the poster I created based on Carsten's inspiration and humbled by the many questions I'm asked by people from all over the world. In some of the countries they represent, millions of people are infected and affected by HIV/AIDS, but have little or no access to the medications that are readily available in the U.S.

From the beginning, when the gay community stepped up to fight the war against AIDS, the message was about empowerment. Most of the questions I'm asked at this conference are not so much about the "Do Not Enter" group I'm speaking about, but more about wanting a deeper understanding of empowerment.

Outside the conference center, I run into protestors urging pharmaceutical companies to give poor countries access to their drugs. That's why the conference was called 'Access for All.' Other countries somehow are not getting access to AIDS medications. I truly understand what the protesters are doing here and I would join them if I could, but I'm not allowed.

I have the opportunity to speak with many people who, like me, are holding small meetings in their communities to help fulfill the current needs of people with HIV/AIDS. I leave feeling empowered, thinking "now is the time to challenge the governments, the pharmaceutical companies and the activists to come to the table and work together for the common good of all people living with HIV/AIDS. The systems in place are like a constant tug of war. The Bush Administration is angry because the activists yell and scream and cause a scene, but that's necessary to get people to listen.

Kofi Annan, Secretary General of the United Nations, said it best: "AIDS is a weapon of mass destruction."

Dr. David Reddy of Basil, Switzerland, and my crew of security people take me to the Global Village to meet Father Joe, Sophie Van Den Bergh, and the children of the Mercy Center. This is one of the many organizations I speak of that performs little miracles every day. My favorite time at the conference is when all the little children of the AIDS orphanage run by the Mercy Center shower me with hugs. These are God's innocent children who lost both parents to AIDS and who may or may not be living with the virus himself or herself.

The miracles keep happening even after the conference ends. Bob and I are on our way home from the conference; we fly from Bangkok to Singapore and then home to Newark Airport from there. On our short flight from Bangkok, I am sitting in an isle seat, and Bob is sitting on my left. I see a man coming down the isle who catches my eye because he is ruggedly handsome but very tough looking. He sits down in the isle seat right across from me. My first impression is he does not look like he wants to be bothered, so I try not to look at him too much. The way it turns out he wants to talk to me. He looks at me and nods and I say hello. When he responds I can hear his Russian accent.

He asks, "Are you from the U.S.?"

I answer, "Yes, from New Jersey."

"So what brings you here to this part of the world?" he asks.

At first I am a little nervous to say why I was there, but I decide to be proud so I responded, "I was here for the International AIDS Conference."

He asks, are you a doctor?"

I was going to say "No, I'm just a nurse" but I catch myself. I sort of throw back my shoulders a little and said, "No I'm a nurse and I was one of the presenters at the conference."

I give him a very short version of what my role at the conference was, and especially glowed as I speak about the children of the Mercy Center. For a short while after I finish, he becomes silent as if he is in deep thought.

Suddenly he says to me, "Can I tell you something in confidence?"

I said, "Sure, of course you can."

I almost fall out into the aisle when he tells me he is gay and his partner lives in Singapore. They have a good friend who is HIV+ and has no access to medication and they really cannot tell a soul that this friend has HIV. Since the whole conference was about 'Global Access,' I immediately think to give him my card. I am already planning in my head to talk to my friends Jaime and Jesus at AID for AIDS, surely they will find a way to get his friend into treatment. I will not use the name of my new friend from the flight to Singapore nor will I ever be able to reveal the name of his friend due to issues of confidentiality. But I can say this, his friend was able to get on treatment and my Russian friend and his partner have since moved to Sydney, Australia. We have remained the best of friends since then and his friend is living a healthy life and thriving. Just because we were, 'Talkin About It!'

When I return from the conference, no one is more excited to see me than my friend Trevor. He feels great, he says, and he's enjoying an increase in T-Cells and a lower viral load, while living his life to the fullest.

Trevor goes to every conference we are invited to attend, and he tells everyone about what his new medication is doing for him. We are on tour, getting invited to group meetings all over the Tri-State area and beyond. I have been invited to meetings in London, Milan, and Glasgow to do presentations and empower-ment talks. This allows us to train nurses all over the world who then teach patients how to self-inject medication, and life can go on for many who think their lives are soon over. This is not my work alone, either. This effort takes teams of people. "Each one, teach one."

One day I'm working an early clinic at NJCRI. Our research assistant, who is usually very competent, knows she is supposed to stock the cabinets with test tubes and carriers the day before. Protocol says when you draw blood on a study patient, you are supposed to roll the test-tube in bubble wrap, stick it into a carry container and take it to the lab and then, wearing gloves, open it carefully to spin the blood. This day she doesn't do what she is supposed to do.

I perform my routine, and open the cabinet to get the car-rier container and the cabinet is empty. I have to transport the blood-filled test tubes without a carrier. It is a federal offense to leave HIV blood in tubes on the counter in your exam room unattended. It's also unsafe to carry blood tubes in your hand to take them to the lab. I choose the lesser of two evils and grab the blood tubes. I'm in too much of a rush, and a little angry with myself for not checking prior to the clinic like I usually do. I drop the test tubes; they shatter when they hit the floor.

I'm wearing gloves and no blood spills on me, but I call for help. We then clean the spill using the proper HAZMAT protocol.

It has come to a point at NJCRI that too many changes are happening: a new manager, new department head, new CFO – and little mishaps are going on all around me. For instance, money seems to be missing from the certificates we give out for study visits. I was becoming very frustrated working in this type of environment. I am proactive and progressive in everything I do in life.

I think I know who is stealing and I keep it to myself until someone suggests I took it. I tell the new manager whom I think is taking the cash and she doesn't believe me.

Although I really enjoy all the education I am doing with Fuzeon and the empowerment groups as well as the skills labs and HIV lectures at Christ Hospital School of Nursing, the times are too turbulent at NJCRI.

I talk it through with Bob and we decide I should leave NJCRI to become a consultant.

I hand in my resignation on November 29 and give a month's notice. During this time, I complete all my research responsibilities and leave on good terms. Dr. Perez wishes me well and tells me he's sad to see me go. I tell him he is the best physician I have ever worked for. He quickly corrects me: worked *with* Dominick, not for. We are partners in this fight.

On December 12, the International Free and Accepted Modern Masons (IFAMM) and the Order of the Eastern Star, Chapter Azure 215 honor me with the Making a Difference Award. However, for Positive Connection, 2004 has not been an easy year. We have lost three members: Tanji, Carsten and Joe, all members of our empowerment group.

# I Am the Boss of Me

My role as a consultant is a break in routine for me. For the first time in my life I am self-employed. I have no time card to punch, no receptionist to schedule appointments, no co-workers to chat with by the water cooler and no boss to hand me a paycheck every two weeks. I do it all myself. I make calls to clinics, ASOs (AIDS

Service Organizations), hospitals and to any group looking for an education/empowerment session. I also continue to check in on all the AIDS support groups and it frees up a little time to clean out the church basement to build a thrift shop down there. The plan is to employ the members of Positive Connection who are not working and give back to the church for the use of the space.

We apply for a grant given by the Episcopal Ministries of the Newark Diocese, and other grants that are available to AIDS Service Organizations. Trevor and I are also doing a course/demonstration for all the new hires at Roche Pharmaceuticals in Nutley, New Jersey. Trevor wants to continue talking about the injectable medication that gives him a new life.

The company sets up forums with nurses and physicians and sometimes, I facilitate the groups. We have forums like this all over the country and I am even called to Canada and England to help nurses set up empowerment groups in their countries. We do one fundraiser every month for Positive Connection, and the group members take full responsibility in running them. It's all working like a charm.

With my new job as a consultant I'm also able to be more involved in ANAC-NJ (Association of Nurses in AIDS Care - New Jersey) Chapter.

At Positive Connection we choose a slogan 'We will thrive in 2005,' to live up to this coming year. Positive Connection now has four groups running. Our regular Monday group at St. John's in Union City and our three focus groups: the gay group in Newark facilitated by Robert; the Fuzeon Group at Broadway House facilitated by Trevor, Karen and I; and the new group for Spanish-speaking people with HIV/AIDS run by Susan Garcia, a social worker at the Peter Ho Clinic at St. Michael's Medical Center. We are preparing for a banner year.

May is always the time of year that Positive Connections awards a scholarship and this year it goes to John M, who is in the process of writing a book of poetry he hopes to publish. Although John is elated to receive the scholarship, he's not happy to know the Thrift Shop we were planning to open will not come to fruition. The building is almost 100 years old and there are issues with flooding, so we have to postpone the opening day to sometime in August.

Trevor, who is a plumber by trade, is trying to help me figure out why we are having so many water problems. He says he can fix it, but I won't allow him to do the work because of the risks involved with dirty water. Trevor is determined to help, so he snakes out the drain from the outside all the way into the building while I am at work doing a presentation.

After testing out the drainage system a few times, Trevor thinks it's working well so we plan a late August opening date.

We take the time after that to set everything up. We had to paint, put up shelving units and collect items for sale. Then we get hit with two hurricanes in one month. The basement floods again and it's really bad this time.

On Sunday, the day after the intended opening, I make an announcement in church that we are not going to open the Thrift Shop and I overhear a woman who was treasurer of the church council, say, "Good! I did not want that riff-raff coming up and down the alley all week anyway."

I rarely get angry, but I became irate at this woman's insensitivity. The minister and the Vestry Warden are standing right there, and see how upset I am by her bigoted and racist remark, but they do nothing. I blow a gasket and storm out of the church.

When I get home I'm hyperventilating. That woman's hateful words cause a huge problem. Bob calls Florence to help calm me down. Robert would have come as well but he is having issues with the new medications he's taking.

The worst part is that Trevor has contracted bacterial pneumonia likely from the work we were doing in the basement when it flooded.

Positive Connection also has to endure the financial burden of paying back the grant because the project does not come to fruition.

I decide that because that woman is a known homophobe, and a racist, I cannot keep my group at that church. I also can no longer stay at the church. So I withdraw my group, and my weekly support, and I decide to take a break from Positive Connection for a while.

The lesson here is, learn and know up front that before you do anything for anyone, there will always be someone who opposes it or tries to ruin a good plan.

What I learn from this tough lesson is that I still have to walk my own path, set my own goals and love my enemies despite how much it hurts, or who that enemy is. This is my journey, and no one else's to walk. As long as I am empowering others to live better lives I will continue to walk as many miles as it takes.

Empowerment meetings are held in my home until we secure a new meeting place. This time I say 'no churches' but news travels fast. Two weeks later I receive a letter from St. Peter's Episcopal Church in Clifton, New Jersey, asking if we wanted to use the facility there to do a support group. With Trevor in the hospital and getting worse every day I did not even think to respond at that time.

# Our Hero

When I first met Trevor he was frail and very ill. His nurse practitioner asked if I would be able to get him into the T-20-305 clinical trial for the medication Fuzeon, which was approved by the FDA in March 2003. We were given three slots and I had already randomized my three patients. I called and wrote letters to Roche and Trimeris asking if they would give me three more slots. I already had Trevor and two others lined up for the trial drug, and thank God, it was approved.

As time went on Trevor started to feel better and his numbers improved. We became more than just nurse and patient. we became good friends. At the time, Trevor told me he had not disclosed his HIV status to anyone except his family; his wife, his mom, and his brother, all three of whom I met at clinic visits. Trevor helped me educate others about how to use Fuzeon.

At the end of the year, representatives from LA Bruell Production Company ask if I would host a video shoot in my Newark, NJ home. Along with Trevor, Nurse Karen and Ira who is also taking the medication, we simulate a Fuzeon 'Do Not Enter' Empowerment Group. We hope to launch a National Empowerment Group Network throughout the country, and perhaps throughout the world, to benefit patients on Fuzeon.

L.A. Bruell contacted us to do a revision for the educational video. Trevor and I go to New York City for the filming. Trevor is so proud whenever we show the video at our 'Do Not Enter' empowerment groups.

We become an educational duo. Through this venue Trevor begins to feel more comfortable with his status and with disclosing it. His family remains his top priority, but his love of helping others in the same situation just keeps growing. We share many stories on our one-day trips and occasional overnights. He always speaks of his wife and family most affectionately on these trips. Trevor becomes a member of Positive Connection and he co-facilitates the Wednesday group at Broadway House with Nurse Karen. Trevor works hard for the group's success and for the completion of the thrift shop. This was not to be, simply because there are too many haters in the world, even ones that go to church.

Trevor passes away on September 29. We receive letters from people in seven different states where we presented. We also received notes from several members of the group; Lucy and Ned from the production company in New York City, even our Roche friends in Basil, Switzerland Neil and Janet send condolences. Trevor is our champion and our hero and his memory will live on.

# Each One, Teach One

Robert, Shamea, and Roro are speakers with the Positive Connection Speakers Bureau. Every time there is a chance for one of them to share their message, they are there. Roro tells her story about how she became aware of her HIV diagnosis while pregnant and how her fiancé died leaving her alone in Florida. Roro always ends by saying how she is doing today. With her medications, her family support, and the empowerment she feels after group meetings, she knows she will be a long-term survivor.

Shamea tells how when she was first diagnosed her T-Cell count was zero and her viral load was one million. This is not a good prognosis. She goes on to say how grateful she is to God, family, and her group. "Positive Connection has helped me to cope with this disease by empowering me to focus on the positive aspects of my life, rather than taking pity on myself for being sick,"

In the past, Robert never saw himself talking about his life in front of large groups of people. His presentation is usually the longest and perhaps the most convincing when it comes to change. While everyone has to deal with changes in their lives, probably many times, Robert created the change he wanted to see. Pretty much from his deathbed Robert set out to beat AIDS by changing his life from a drug-and-alcohol-fueled life to a new one working toward optimal health.

Diagnosed in 1988 and living through life-threatening anemia from AZT, Robert became empowered once he was invited to join Positive Connection. He has a take-charge attitude and even began facilitating his own Positive Connection sponsored group for gay men, to share what he learned with others.

"Each one, Teach One," he says, "I used to live with the shame, stigma and shock of it all, but now I live with a creative spirit, writing poetry, and a column in the newsletter *Talkin' About It!* Being involved in Positive Connection has been the most beneficial move I have ever made in my life. I am inspired now to teach others to be empowered and to live a non-toxic healthy lifestyle."

# Go Fund Me

In early April, I invited Sally Deering, an award-winning reporter and syndicated columnist, to attend the first anniversary party of Positive Connection. After the party, Sally says she went home to do her taxes and was looking for the little red box to make a tax donation to an AIDS charity, but there wasn't any.

Since Bob always does my taxes I have no idea what she is talking about. Sally explains on the phone: "The Children's Trust Fund, the Wildlife Fund and many others have a space asking anyone receiving a tax refund if they would like to donate any amount of their tax return to one or more of those organizations," she says.

We both agree something should be done about it; and we go to work. Sally does most of the investigating and I vow my support 100%. Sally calls back right after calling the New Jersey Treasurer's Office. They told Sally that the charities appear on the New Jersey State Tax forms only with the approval of the State Assembly, then the Senate, and then with final approval by the Governor. I tell Sally this might be easier than we thought.

State Assemblywoman Joan Quigley is a friend and neighbor and I know she will support this. Sally knows State Senator Berne Kenny who will also support it. Assemblywoman Quigley and Senator Kenny both receive calls from Sally and they promise to work together quickly to propose a Bill in the Assembly.

Assemblywoman Quigley also says to Sally "I promise this Bill will be written up by June 1st," and it is. The following week Sally tells the story in her syndicated column. She wrote, *"Think of the money we could raise for AIDS programs like Positive Connection, just by marking a little box for the AIDS Services Fund."* And her final paragraph: *"On my way to the post office to mail my tax form, I passed a line of people buying lottery tickets. If all it takes is a dollar and a dream to win the lottery, just think of what a dollar donation could win in the fight against AIDS."*

The AIDS Services Fund Bill S-340 passes unanimously in the Senate Health Committee on June 19, and it continues to pass through other committees. Four months later we find out it is stalled in the Senate Budget and Appropriations Committee. It was time to take action.

The members of Positive Connection send petition forms out to every church, AIDS organization, our family and friends. We stand outside supermarkets getting as many signatures as possible. Within one month I send more than 2000 signatures to State Senator Robert Littell, a Republican from Sussex County. The new date for the Senate Budget and Appropriations Committee to vote is October 19 and Bill S-340 passes unanimously. We are hopeful for a quick vote in the Senate and General Assembly, as is the process in the State of New Jersey. The final vote is the Governor's signature.

# 2005
# One More Push

As usual, the New Year is off to a running start. Our biggest challenge is to get Bill S-340 through the Senate and into the Assembly for a vote. This has to be accomplished before June 10 so that the new forms being printed for the 2005 taxes will have "The AIDS Services Fund" included. We find out right after Christmas that Bill S-340 passed in the Senate with a unanimous 40-0 vote.

This is what happens when people take action and let their voices be heard. It is now in the Assembly and Republican Chairperson, Charlotte Vandervalk needs to hear our voices as well. On January 15, we begin a letter-writing campaign. By now this is way bigger than Sally, me, and Positive Connection.

Every church and AIDS organization supporting the Bill now called A-1867 sends letters and signs petitions. Bill A-1867 has to get through the Assembly Budget Committee and the Ways and Means Committee before going before the General Assembly for a vote.

President George W. Bush takes office on January 20, 2001, and chooses New Jersey Governor Christine Todd Whitman to head up the U.S. Environmental Protection Agency, so Acting Governor Donald DeFrancisco takes over.

The Bill passes the General Assembly with a unanimous vote of 78 to 0 and Acting Governor Donald DeFrancisco signs it just in time for next April's tax forms.

Governor DeFrancisco sends a letter to me on State House stationary thanking me for my participation, and Sally Deering got one too, along with a wonderful write up in the *Jersey Journal* the next day. At Positive Connection's Anniversary and Awards Dinner, we give Sally Deering the Jorge Perez Memorial Award for her work helping people and families affected by HIVAIDS.

# Eight

## 2006
## Flower Child

Dr. Diana Finkle, a wonderful doctor I met at Saint Michael's Medical Center when she was a resident at the AIDS clinic with Dr. Perez and Dr. Slim, calls me out of the blue. Knowing I have experience running support groups, she says on the phone: "I have four AIDS patients here in Clifton and there are no support groups for them. Can you start one? I'll let you use my waiting room Wednesday afternoons."

I take her up on it.

One of the Clifton group's nicest members was Ms. Ruby, a feisty 70-something. Ms. Ruby is a force to be reckoned with, and perhaps the bravest woman I have ever met. Her son or granddaughter always takes her to the group meeting every week. Ms. Ruby, like everyone else, shares her story about how she was infected by her husband who died years before. She never blames him or says one bad word against him in group.

We all love Ms. Ruby's spirit. She says things like, "If I can do it, why can't you?" She causes everyone in the group – including me – to rethink the possibilities. In a sense, Ms. Ruby is the inspiration that brings all our groups together and gives Positive

Connection the jumpstart it needs to keep providing the services we have been providing these last 10 years.

The other three members of the group listen to Ms. Ruby more than they listen to me, which is great because all I have to do is sit and make sure the conversations are focused and on point.

About two months after we began, we now have seven members. Members from the other groups want to join the Clifton group, too.

Another standout member in our Clifton support group is Alana, a 65-year-old Latina. At first she did not want to come to group, but could not say 'no' to Dr. Finkle. (I don't think anyone can say 'no' to Dr. Finkle, she is so sweet.) In fact, the first time she is supposed to come to group, Alana sends her daughter in her place.

We are all in a circle in Dr. Finkle's waiting room, and this young woman starts out by using a false name. "Hello everyone, I'm Lorraine and I have HIV and Dr. Finkle is my doctor, and she suggested I come to this group." she says.

But when everybody makes her feel at ease and at home, she can't keep up the lie any longer, and blurts out: "Alright everyone, I'm very sorry. I don't have HIV. I hope you don't kick me out of this group. I'm sorry."

"It's okay, you can come for the learning experience," I tell her.

"Now I really feel bad," she says. "You see, my mother and my daughter are sitting in the car outside waiting for me. My mother has HIV and she sent me here to check things out."

I look around the room and my jaw is not the only one hitting the floor. She continues, "my mother thinks she won't fit in because everybody will be young, but you're all old."

She quickly apologizes, "I didn't mean to say that!"

She was right though. We have Robert who's 65, Ms. Ruby is 72, I'm in my 50s, Ron is in his 50s, and Raymond just rounded 40 – and he's the youngest.

I look at her and I ask, "Your mother's in the car? Well, go downstairs, get her and bring her up here with your daughter."

Alana and her granddaughter walk in a few minutes later. She then sends her daughter and granddaughter back downstairs because she doesn't want her granddaughter, who is 8, to know she has HIV. She's bawling her eyes out, now, and the group spends the next 30 minutes drying Alana's tears. We all agree that next week will be all about her.

The following week, Alana attends the meeting. When she sits down, she tells us how she got AIDS from her husband who died a couple years back. Her daughter, who is divorced, had a toe amputated because of diabetes and now the doctors are deciding whether to take the foot, too. And Alana's young granddaughter doesn't know how sick her mother and grandmother really are.

Alana, like Ms. Ruby, attends the Clifton support group every week; they soon became great friends and a support system for each other.

It's Alana's birthday and before group that night, Ms. Ruby calls and asks if she can pick up flowers for Alana. I tell her it's a great idea. At the support group, we have a birthday cake for Alana and give her a beautiful bouquet of flowers. She starts to cry.

"No one ever gave me flowers," she says.

Can you imagine?

Alana has had HIV for ten years, although she was infected by her husband, she never says a bad thing about him. Never.

She reveals in the group that he was abusive to her and yet, she upholds his memory. Alana lives in the tight Latino community of Patterson, NJ and tells no one about her diagnosis. She once mentioned in the group that one of her neighbors came up and said to her, in Spanish, "Alana, the guy in apartment 3B has AIDS. You stay away from him. Don't go near him or you will catch it."

She tells us that before she came to the group, her response would have been different. She would have said, "Yes, I won't go near him." But now that's changed. Now she would say, "I know you can't catch AIDS from talking. So don't be afraid"

So now, Alana's educating others in her community and standing up for herself. This is exactly what empowerment groups are meant to do.

We start getting too big for Dr. Finkle's waiting room. That's when I remember that when we were at St. John's in Union City, I sent a letter about World AIDS Day to all the Episcopal churches in New Jersey and three responded. One of those churches wrote back saying we could use their facilities to run a support group if needed, that church was St. Peter's in Clifton. Knowing my history of running groups in a church, I had to decide if I wanted to do it again.

I bring it up at our next Board meeting, and we search for alternatives, but there seems to be nothing else available but St. Peter's, a few blocks from Dr. Finkle's office. We realize that in order for the group to keep going, we have to keep the meetings local for Dr. Finkle's patients to attend. A week later I sign a contract with St. Peter's. Father Peter DeFranco was pleased to be able to house us there.

When I think of flowers I think of all the special occasions where we would give or receive them. I also think of my life and how flowers and flower shops were always intertwined like when

I was eleven years old working in the flower shop for Mr. Delia. I think of the many times on Valentine's Day that I have given flowers or received them. I think of Dawn's flower shop where I got one of my three pushes into the field of nursing. Last I think of all the beautiful Brides and Grooms carefully choosing the perfect flower arrangements for their special day.

# 1997
# Member of the Wedding

It was the beginning of May, Bob and I returned from a quick get-away weekend. A few days earlier a message was left on our answering machine from a nurse colleague, who runs a support group for people with AIDS.

This wonderful Nurse was a pioneer in AIDS Care long before I became an AIDS nurse, and she probably did several groups in the early days when it was called GRID. Unlike non-nurses who lead groups, Eileen has hands-on experience with the needs of her group members. She's my friend and a role model.

"Hi Dominick, it's Eileen," she began, and then got right to it. "The family of one of my patients made a request, and the first person I thought of was you."

She went on to say that one of her patients; a support group member David G. had a brother who was getting married in less than a month. His family needed a professional to help David get ready to be his brother's Best Man at the wedding, and she wanted to know as soon as possible if I would be willing to do that for the family, and how much I would charge.

I spoke to Bob that evening during dinner and he said we definitely did not have plans for that weekend and would not make any. I called Eileen and told her I would do it under one condition, I would not accept payment. She said she would pass along my phone number and thanked me for saying yes.

Minutes later, I received a call from Mrs. G., David's mom. She sounded like a wonderful person and terrific mother who was concerned about her son's health and well-being – a refreshing change from the many friends I have known through the years whose parents disowned them for being gay, even after finding out they were living with AIDS. Even then, they would not take them in and care for them. Hard to believe, but true.

Mrs. G. and I had a long talk. She told me David is her best friend, her strength and even her fashion consultant. This family knew how important this day was for David's brother, Martin and his bride-to-be, Patty, and special to David as well. They also knew they would all be extremely busy, as most families are during a wedding, and they wanted someone, preferably a medical professional, to be there for David.

While on the phone, "I told Mrs. G. I would do anything she needed me to do and if I had to, I'd do it in heels." She laughed so heartily. I liked her immediately, but I told Mrs. G. I would not accept payment, and I would be there to help David for the entire evening.

Mrs. G. said, "I can understand you're not wanting to get paid, and I still disagree with that, but I will honor that request. However, you will sit at the table right next to David, and you will be a member of our family for the entire evening."

I liked her even more than before.

It was June 13, the day of the wedding, and I showered, shaved and dressed. In my usual style I arrived at the hotel early, sat in my car and said a prayer that I would be able to accomplish everything that was requested of me with kindness and compassion.

I walked into the hotel, went to the Concierge desk and asked for David's room. I took the elevator to the 7th floor and Mr. and Mrs. G. greeted me at the door. They both looked stunning in their wedding attire. David was in bed, showered and attentive. Tall like my Bob, slender, and handsome with beautiful gray/green eyes.

I walked over to his bed and introduced myself. We spoke for a few minutes and he was delightful. I could also see that he was in pain. Living with AIDS, David had peripheral neuropathy, which is tingling sensation in the lower legs that is so painful it can cause an inability to walk or stand.

I began to help David get dressed. Because he was in such terrible pain – even the act of putting on socks was going to be painful – I stretched each sock over my hands and then peeled them onto his feet, trying my best not to rub the socks or my hands on his skin. David gave a sigh of relief.

Dressed and ready to head to the hall where the ceremony was to take place, David looked at me as we approached the door and said, "I really appreciate your gentle kindness." I leaned in, kissed him on the forehead and said, "I feel honored to do this for you and your family David. My only concern is that I might trip."

"Don't worry, if you do, we can get you a wheelchair, too."

We both laughed and off we went. I did not know this man two hours and already I loved him like a best friend. Intelligent, good-looking, funny – those are all the qualities I saw in Bob when we first met 11 years ago in 1986. It's no wonder I liked David so much. He reminded me of the man I love.

David's brother Martin looked very handsome in his black tuxedo; and his bride Patty looked absolutely beautiful. I stood with David at the altar as they exchanged vows. And before I knew it the ceremony was over.

We went into the ballroom for the reception. Just as Mrs. G. promised, I was seated next to David at the family table. The food was great and my conversation with David, and his family even better. We learned so much about each other in such a short amount of time. By the end of the reception I felt I had known him my whole life.

My very last task of the evening was to take David to his room, help him undress and tuck him in bed. Before we went up, David said to his mom, "I wish I had met Dominick a long time ago."

I felt the same way about him.

I said my goodbyes to Mr. and Mrs. G, Martin and Patty, and took David upstairs to his suite. It was about 10 pm and he was very tired. Not me. I was too happy and excited to be a part of this wonderful family event. I got him into his nightwear, and tucked him in.

"Dominick," he said, "Where have you been all my life?"

We laughed together one more time.

"Thank you," he said.

"No, thank you, David."

I leaned over and kissed his forehead again. "Goodnight David, I hope to see you real soon."

He smiled. I turned out the light and let myself out.

When I got home, I wanted to tell Bob all about David and the night we had. Poor Bob! It was 11 o'clock at night and all he wanted to do was go to sleep. He graciously stayed up with me for as long as he could. I was about to take off my suit jacket and went to empty my pockets when there was a check written out to Project H.E.L.P. And a note from Mrs. G: *Thank you for being the amazing person you are.*

I called Mrs. G. a few days later to thank her. I asked how my new buddy David was doing. She told me that he used to have good and bad days, but now they were mostly bad. I asked if it would be okay to visit him and she said, "David would love that."

August 20 was David's 34th birthday and I called to wish him Happy Birthday. Mrs. G. told me David was in the hospital and they would be celebrating his birthday there with a cake.

On September 27, three months after his brother's wedding, David succumbed to AIDS and passed away. A few years later, when his niece Tory was in Middle School, her teacher asked the class to write an essay about a tragedy that occurred in the family. Tori wrote her essay about her Uncle David. I'm adding it here just the way she wrote it; with the A+ she earned for writing from the heart.

# My Journey as an AIDS Nurse

Tony Pierson                    March 12, 200
Writing / Period-6             Ms. Ofalt

## Tragedie in my Family

My Uncle David was a big part of our lives. He died unfortunatly from a disease called AIDS on September 27, 1997. He had been very ill for a while and there was no medication we could give to him to make him 100% better. My family was supposed to go to a wedding in Colorado but didn't want to leave him behind, especially not knowing what would occur with him in those days they were gone. My uncle told them there was no use in not going because they couldn't help him anyway. Someone needed to stay behind with him however, so my grandpa (my uncle's father) did the job with no complaints. Everyone was off to the wedding to have a good time. Then in the early morning before the wedding my grandma got a call from my grandpa saying that David had passed on, but my grandma knew as soon as she heard the first ring. Everyone was so upset but couldn't just leave Colorado because of the wedding. They went through the day sadly and decided it would be better to tell the bride and groom after their big day. That night they all left, and couldn't believe that god finally had him. Not that they didn't love him, but he was suffering, he was something no person couldn't call special. A few days after we had the wake and burial. My mother was extremly close to David and I have never ever seen her cry as much as she did during the LAST time she would see him before the casket was closed for good. She was histerical. The family think

219

My uncle David wanted to die when nobody was around, because he picked his day to die. This is proven because my mother's birthday is September 9th and my uncle David gave her a card, and written on it was: co 27 in handwriting that was jagged and not very clear to read. That meant that he would pass away when everyone was in Colorado on the 27th. Only my grandpa was with him at the house, and David waited to die until he saw his father one final time. My grandpa left David's side for only about one (1) minute to put some coffee on, and when he came back, my uncle was dead. I imagine him now however in Heaven as an angel. I know that my uncle David watches over me and I like to think of him as my guardian angel. I think if anyone in the world has a fear of dying – they shouldn't, because David is there and I'm sure he would make anyone feel comfortable. David loved Pooh Bear and everytime I see it I think of him. My whole family misses him, but he knows we will always love him no matter where he is.

### ✻ BONUS ↝ EXTRA CREDIT ✻

If anyone besides a person knew there was something wrong during the tragedie it was his cute dog named Tom Sawyer. I remember everyone was crying and he would moan. Also, he acted like he was missing something (his owner) and he was correct. Everyone could tell Sawyer missed David. Shortly after my uncle's death we had to put the dog to sleep because he was old and sick. When we did this we put a picture of David in front of Sawyer so the last thing he saw would be David. All we know now is David Roman Gordenovich is with Sawyer.

The Soul Would have No Rainbow if The Eyes had No Tear
MINQUASS PROV

I did not know David a long time, but we shared something very meaningful that brought me into his life and his family. With David's passing – his life cut short by AIDS – I am reminded that death is God's will, not ours, or we would hold onto our loved ones and never let go.

# 2006
# Remember and Celebrate

World AIDS Day is commemorated every year on December 1st and once again our list of people who died from AIDS has grown. At Positive Connection's annual Memorial Tribute, we honor the family members, group members and friends we lost, as well as Jorge and David G. who never had the opportunity to attended one of our group meetings, but we feel they are a part of our Positive Connection family in spirit. The reason we commemorate the lives of these individuals every year to always remind us that they were important pieces of our quilt of life.

We must always remember to never become complacent with this illness or any other or the cycle will start over again. While fewer people in the United States are dying from AIDS because of the advancements we have made, there are still 50 thousand new cases of AIDS every year, mostly the younger people who did not live and learn the way we did in the 1980's. We must give tribute every year to the brave people of our LGBTQ community.

Meanwhile, Positive Connection's Scholarship Committee is always busy deciding who will receive the award each year. Roro wrote a beautiful letter telling the committee about her life of missed educational opportunities, and how she wants to go to school to learn computers. We do not want one more opportunity to slip by her, so Roro was awarded the scholarship to pay for a computer and school tuition. Our scholarship program at Positive Connection has become a very important part of what we try to accomplish.

In the beginning when GRID took a grip on the gay community many of our lesbian sisters stepped up to the plate. This was such an historic time when our LGBTQ community came together as one unit to fight the political system that held us back and made us second class citizens. Gay men were losing their jobs, apartments, and in many cases, even their families for being gay and or having AIDS.

This is why Positive Connection chose to name our scholarship for David G. David was a gifted young gay man who fought bravely to the end. I had the pleasure of knowing him for a very short time, however it is David's family I boast about now. You know, 'They' say you cannot choose your family and that is true. But if we could pick those we would want as our family, this family would be a number one choice of anyone who ever knew them. This entire family stood by their gay son, brother, uncle, and friend through every pain for several years. To me they are and continue to be 'The Gold Star Family' of HIV/AIDS.

## What Have We Learned?

At this time, Positive Connection members and I attend three major AIDS conferences: The National Conference on African Americans and AIDS in Philadelphia, which I attend with Miss Florence; the Latino Conference on AIDS in Miami that I go to with Reymundo; and the 16th International Aids Conference in Toronto, Canada, which I attend alone, paying my travel and hotel expenses out-of-pocket.

# My Journey as an AIDS Nurse

At the African Americans and AIDS conference Florence and I attend in Philadelphia, the Rev. Jesse Jackson is the Keynote Speaker and gives an amazing speech. At the end of it, Florence looks at me and says, "I think we just did church." Trevor and I were also there to give an injection demonstration that was well attended.

At the Latino AIDS Conference, actor Erik Estrada (one of my childhood heart throbs) gives the Keynote address. At this conference many of the sessions deal with Latinas who are marginalized by their husbands and families. Latina women need to take a more visible role in the prevention and treatment of HIV in their lives and the lives of their children. Something needs to be done to break the stigma women seem to face. Erik Estrada hammered that home, and yes his pants were just as tight as they were when he was on the show C.H.I.P. S. in the 1970's.

My favorite speaker at the AIDS conference in Miami is Dr. Ivan Melendez from Ponce, Puerto Rico. Dr. Melendez not only addresses Latinos and AIDS, he addresses all people who are marginalized and stigmatized by AIDS after 25 years since the first outbreak. He speaks about the U.S. Presidential Election coming up in 2008, and urges us all to listen carefully about what the candidates say about AIDS – from the primaries to the conventions up to Election Day. He talks passionately about the subject and I am awestruck. I must meet him; and I did. I was trying to see if I could arrange a talk in Puerto Rico and get to see the Perez family at the same time.

I attend the Toronto AIDS conference as a volunteer, not a speaker. I also meet some really wonderful people; as I did in Thailand.

This conference, like most others, brings together scientists, physicians, nurses, and allied health professionals who outline where we are and where we are headed in the war on AIDS. At the conference, there is a separate area known as the Global Village where non-medical participants can gather to share their ways of fighting HIV/AIDS in their communities. This is where I'm stationed; right where I feel most comfortable.

As a conference delegate in Thailand, I presented my work globally rather than to my local community. In Toronto, I'm with the people. As a volunteer, my job is to greet conference attendees, work the information booth and the PWA (People With AIDS) lounge, where my duties are to be sure they there relaxing, taking their medications and have refreshments and snacks to nosh on. We even give foot massages. I think I enjoy that day the most. When I have time off, I visit vendors and others I know from Thailand, and make new contacts.

While my colleagues are busy talking about the newest treatments and scientific discoveries like microbicides and vaccines and the money or lack thereof needed to fight this pandemic worldwide, 2,000 volunteers help it run smoothly.

Noticeably missing from the conference are President George W. Bush and the Canadian Prime Minister Stephen Harper. On hand to help the cause are Bill and Melinda Gates and President Bill Clinton. As I walk across the bridge from the Global Village to the vendors' area, security stops a group of us in front of a bank of elevators because a dignitary needs to get through. The doors open and there right in front of me, is President Clinton. With the Secret Service surrounding him, he walks straight to me and shakes my hand. Then he continues down the line, shaking hands and greeting the conference-goers. I feel a proud American moment, something I have not had since 9/11.

The clear favorite of the conference is United Nations Special Envoy, Ambassador Stephen Lewis. He is perhaps the most vocal of the 40,000 attendees in the auditorium. Lewis blasts President Bush and Canada's Prime Minister Stephen Harper, saying, "The more we use their actual names the more power we give them." (Neither Bush nor Harper's name is mentioned in the *Ottawa Citizens* newspaper handed out in the Global Village) In his speech, Lewis refers to them as "ignorant world leaders." Lewis also dismisses South Africa's government, which has completely ignored its AIDS epidemic.

"What do they think? It will just go away!" he says to thunderous applause. At a symposium for AIDS Nurses, a nurse from South Africa affirms Lewis' anger toward South Africa's leaders and the toll it takes on AIDS caregivers: "Nurses are the backbone of care in HIV/AIDS," she says," and my backbone is broken."

I have never been more proud of being an AIDS Nurse than this moment when I stand with thousands of other AIDS Nurses bonding in our tears and our commitment to keep up the fight.

This beautiful South African Aids Nurse goes on to say that nurses in South Africa work 24/7 and get paid $300 a month.

After the conference I fly back to New Jersey and my beautiful home in Newark, and tell myself that now, I must practice what I preach.

# Nine

## 2007
## Finding my way back

This year Positive Connection doesn't celebrate with an anniversary party like in years' past. We simply take all the members of each group out to dinner; and give out the annual scholarship award.

Robert has always been a very active guy and as members of the Positive Connection Board of Directors, we spend a lot of time together shopping and running errands for all the groups.

Recently Robert was put on different medication and he is having problems with his legs making him unable to get around as easily as he did before. Despite the fact that he has already been given a scholarship, we decide to give him another one so he can take an art class – something he's wanted to do ever since he was a kid. Robert sent a beautiful letter to the scholarship committee, which was then sent to David's family. Robert worked almost every day on his art and I must say he was pretty good. At our empowerment groups it is all about making people's dreams and wishes come true. Too many opportunities went by the wayside for way too long because even eight years into the new millennium, people with AIDS were discriminated against, for being gay, black, or female, and too many times our discussions in the group had to turn to how will we help each other through it. Once a person is a racist, bigoted hater it is unlikely that they will change. But hate is bad Karma and love is good karma. This is a lesson I share every day. The more people hate, the more you must try to turn that hate into love.

# 1987
# I Can't Tell You Where I'm Going

From the very beginning of our relationship Bob knew my heart – and I knew his. When we got our first apartment together on Montgomery Street in Jersey City, I took him for a tour of the neighborhood. Just up the street was where my friend, Guy worked. I really wish Bob could have met Guy. There was something special about him.

Guy was a wonderful man with GQ looks and a heart of gold. I had known Guy since I was 11. Guy was 19. Even at a young age, I always felt attracted to him although I would never act on this attraction because I was too busy trying to convince myself that I was a ladies man. I never knew Guy was gay until two years ago when I ran into him on Washington Street in Hoboken. Guy told me he was living there in Hoboken, but preparing to move. It was a bit strange how he told me.

"You may never see me again once I give up my apartment," he said.

"Why, where are you going?" I asked.

"I'm not really sure yet," he said. I'm just not going to be here."

I was puzzled, but I really wanted to keep in touch with him, so I told him that Bob and I were moving to Montgomery Street in Jersey City right up the street from where we first met at the auto parts store, and I gave him my number hoping we would stay in touch. We hugged and his last words to me were "be careful out there."

About two years later, I went into the new auto parts shop across the street from the old Montgomery Auto Parts store was, where Guy's sister, Sandy was working. I hesitated to ask Sandy about Guy, but I had to know how he was doing. When Sandy saw me, her eyes started to tear up.

"Hi, how are you?" I asked. "How is your brother, Guy?"

"Guy died on March 21ˢᵗ," she said.

Once again as it happened too many times before, I was grieving the loss of a friend. It was getting to the point that gay men were afraid to ask about someone if they have not heard from them in awhile.

I felt like I had to leave the auto parts store because I was overcome by the news. Before I left, I hugged Sandy and asked her if she would tell me where he was buried. It was Holy Name Cemetery across the street on West Side Avenue.

Filled with sadness over the loss of my dear childhood friend, I walked over to his gravesite. The only thing I could think of to do was to put a rock on his tombstone. I said "Thank you God for putting Guy in my life. Help me to be as kind and generous as he was."

I sat in my car awhile before I could drive home, and I thought about Guy and the hell he must have gone through being gay in the 1960s, 70s, and 80s. The homophobia that permeated our culture and forced so many of us to stay in the closet where it was presumably safe still exists, and we all paid the price.

As I sat there mourning Guy, the thoughts in my head turned to all the gay bashing I took when I came out as a gay man working as a railroad repairman. After 15 years on the job, my managers at South Kearny Railway decided to make my life a living hell.

# My Journey as an AIDS Nurse

I remember there was tremendous growth in the field maintenance department. Railroad repair shops all over the country were closing, repairs to the railroad cars were being done by mobile maintenance repairmen. I was the supervisor of the Northeast Mobile Unit overseeing every rail yard from Portland, Maine, to Alexandria, Virginia. My workload had become very intense. Monthly inspections made in my area had me traveling a lot; meanwhile Bob was busy at NYU working on his MBA.

Bob and I always made our schedules work, but these days I rarely had time to share with him the homophobia I was facing every day at work. Somehow, my manager Mr. K figured out – or found out – I was gay, and he tortured me endlessly to get me to quit my job. I just kept silent and kept working, at first, but the fighter and activist in me began to emerge. My boss could not find a way to fire me because my work ethic was excellent, so he began to exploit my being gay as a tactic to make me quit. It started when we were in Baltimore for a company meeting.

We were at lunch, and during cocktails, our waiter (who I could tell was gay) accidentally spilled something on my manager. I grabbed napkins to help the waiter clean up the spill and Mr. K said to me in a very loud voice, "Don't help him. What are you some kind of faggot?"

Later, at our meeting, two supervisors were teaching me the new computer program that was getting installed system-wide. They were each teaching me different things at the same time and I was confused. One would say hit this button and the other would say no it's this one. When all the mobile van drivers and supervisors came together later that day Mr. K had the floor explaining the program to everyone he looked directly at me and in front of the entire department said, "We are very proud of this program. It makes me as happy as a queer with a dick in his mouth."

I was mortified; everyone else cracked up laughing.

Mr. K then went on to say, "We need to work as a team, only we don't know what team Dominick is on."

That provoked more hateful laughter; and I just couldn't hold back any longer.

"Well, Mr. K, how could you *not* know what team I play for, when you are my coach?"

The laughter at that remark was more like a roar, which prompted Mr. K's boss to call a recess.

There were so many times I had to endure this at meetings and conferences but I would not give in and in my own way gave it right back to him.

And as I sat in my car and cried over the loss of my friend Guy, I vowed that I would never ever allow anyone to gay bash me or anyone else in my presence. No more words like faggot; and no more queers sucking dick jokes. I'm done with this type of blatant discrimination.

This one's for you, Guy.


# 2007
## Condom Man...

I'm working less and less as the year goes on, so in order to keep myself occupied I step up on the 'End AIDS as We Know It' initiative. This was a program supported by the caregivers of Saint Michael's Medical Center and the newly elected Mayor of Newark, NJ Cory Booker. It was time for me to put on my tights and become 'The Condom Man.'

Where I live in Newark, there are sex workers in Branch Brook Park – men and women – who ply their trade in the dense trees and bushes in the park's various sections. So, I drive to a specific spot and call out to them that I'm handing out free condoms so that they will be safe.

"I'm not here to judge you," I say, "I'm here to help you be safe."

I know I can't stop them from putting their health in danger, but I can at least give them a chance to be more conscious of it. I will never know if this was effective but even if it was effective for just one person I would feel accomplished in that mission.

In addition, I decide to supplement my income by teaching people how to use a medication for wasting syndrome called Serostim, which is taken with a needleless injection device called the 'Sero-Jet.' Like I had done with injectable medications in the past I was now given yet another opportunity to teach patients and nurses by doing patient education programs for them. The two representatives I worked with most often, Liz in New Jersey and Jen in New York were extraordinary in setting these programs up for me. Liz is a nurse and the Jen a nutritionist. Through this teaching I had met many wonderful patients like Lori, Ray, and Chris. I had the honor of meeting and working with some wonderful physicians like Dr. Frank Spinelli in NYC. Terrific opportunities lead to terrific experiences in life to anyone who is willing to put their God given talents out there.

By the end of 2007 the economy started to tank and companies were no longer able to hire me and I had to rethink what my next role, as an AIDS Nurse would be.

# Grandma speaks from the grave...

Meanwhile, the ANAC National Conference is coming up and I have to be there because I am the incoming president of the New Jersey Chapter. I pay my conference fees and secure my hotel room in Orlando.

A few days before the conference begins my friend Angelo, a clinical trial nurse at Jacoby Medical Center in The Bronx, calls me to ask if I have a room for the conference. He was so busy at work that he forgot to book a room and they were booked solid for the whole week. I tell him I have a room with two beds and that it would be great if we could share because money's a little tight right now.

We meet at the Orlando airport and the first night we sit and talk for hours. When Angelo discovers I'm looking for a job he tells me they have an opening for a research nurse at Jacoby. Since I have research experience, I take him up on the offer, and after the conference I apply for the job. The next day, they call me in for an interview.

At 9:50 am the following Tuesday, I meet Angelo and his boss. The interview goes well and they tell me I'm just the person they're looking for and what the job pays if I accept it. I almost fall off my chair. I choke back my emotions and say, "Sounds great. I'll let you know by Friday."

We shake hands all around and they walk me to the entrance of the hospital. I'm so excited; I barely notice it's raining, no not raining pouring. I buy an umbrella at the gift shop and don't care how much it costs. When I get home it's nearly 3 pm, I get out of my wet clothes, take a hot shower and wait for Bob to come home from work so we can talk about it.

I know I'm going to take the job, but I need to hear Bob's perspective. I also know it will not be easy getting up at 5 am to be in work by 8 am and then leave the Bronx at 4:30 pm and get home about 6:30. I also have to wonder how I will be able to keep Positive Connection's three groups going. The Belleville group runs fine with Robert, but I will not be able to stop by to visit anymore. Nurse Karen runs the Wednesday Fuzeon Group, and the Clifton group will have to close or get a new facilitator.

The next morning, I know what I have to do, I visit Grandma's grave. I always get answers to my questions when I do that. I also go to the Chapel at Christ Hospital.

At the chapel, I write in the spiral notebook about my important decision and what should I do about the job offer. I leave quietly, and return home. I'm eating lunch and the telephone rings. It's Jeanine Reilly, executive director at Broadway House.

"Dominick" she says, "Broadway House needs you back. I was speaking with Maggie our Nurse Practitioner and she agrees you would be very helpful to her and the staff if you would consider taking this job that just became available. How soon can you come in for the interview?"

She actually had me as soon as she said "Needs you back," I'm stammering, but muster up enough poise to say "How about tomorrow morning?"

"Okay" she says. "10am", right after morning report."

I hang up the phone knowing I have been spiritually guided back to Broadway House. Although the salary Broadway House is offing is substantially less than what Jacoby is offering, I take the job at Broadway House.

I call Angelo and tell him. He says, "Dominick, no hard feelings. I think you made the right decision."

My new job at Broadway House has brought me full circle. I started as an AIDS nurse here in 1994, and I knew I would come back someday.

## 2008
## Mr. President

Being back at Broadway House has led to amazing opportunities for me educating both patients and staff. As president of ANAC-NJ, we had four programs to plan. They were all very successful and well attended. At the end of the year we did a major fund-raiser called "The Red Ribbon Ball" This was a black tie affair enabling us to raise funds for local AIDS organizations.

In November, I attend the National Conference held in Reno, Nevada. I decide to go to a symposium on transgendered people who are HIV-positive. When I get there, I sit next to my friend Bill from D.C. I say to him, "Who is that handsome guy speaking?"

He tells me he is Samuel Laurie, a 'trans-man' who is pretty well known, I was shocked. I listened intently to him speak. Mr. Laurie in one lecture taught me so much about the part of the LGBTQ community I knew least about and today I am a proud Trans-Ally. I really needed this session to broaden my knowledge of the transgendered community so I can be better at my job as nurse liaison. I know a few people who are transgendered and Samuel helped me to become better informed. Afterwards I introduce myself and invite Samuel do two speaking engagements in New Jersey. Samuel turned out to be a great friend to Broadway House, just in time to guide us as we admitted two transgendered patients in one month. A life experience I will never forget and never regret. Proof to me that God's wonders come through in every human being He has created.

## Dream a Little Dream

I'm thinking about the communication section of this Palliative Care Initiative I'm working on and I'm trying to come up with an example of Good Communication at Broadway House. Then, I remember Gary G.

Shortly before Christmas, Gary, a resident at Broadway House, has the idea that he wants to get out of Broadway House and get a job and start living his life again. I remember him asking just about everyone who works here if they could buy him a bowtie. Why in the world does he want a bowtie, I think.

He tells me in no uncertain terms that he is going to use the bowtie for his upcoming job interviews. What I fail to realize is that Gary is communicating his dreams to me and I just was not getting it.

I think we all tried to look for a bowtie for Gary. I know the folks in activities did and I am sure others did as well. I went home the day he asked me and rummaged through my closets and dresser drawers but could not find a bowtie anywhere.

I shrugged it off, thinking tomorrow he won't even remember that he asked for it, but the next day, he did remember, and for the next several days he would ask me every morning. I went to the stores but couldn't find a bowtie. I asked several people and they said the same thing: "don't worry about it."

Fast-forward to Christmas Eve 2008 and I'm on my way to Mass at Saint Peter's Episcopal church in Clifton. I stop at a red light and look to the right. There, on the corner, is a men's clothing store open till 10 pm. I think maybe they'll have a bowtie. I pull over, go inside and they have one black bowtie for $5.

Christmas morning, the bowtie goes into Gary's Christmas stocking. Well, once he saw it, nothing else mattered much to him. He could now start going on interviews for the job he was determined to get. There was fireman, social worker, and at one point, he even looked into becoming a lawyer. Gary actually got on the phone and interviewed for these positions.

So what does all this have to do with communication? Well, I believe Gary was trying to communicate his dream to all of us. Maybe he knew he was dying. Maybe he didn't. But the one thing he did know was that he was going to find a job if it was the last thing he did and he didn't let us stop him even when we doubted him.

I know I dropped the ball on this one, only seeing the impossibility of bringing this dream to fruition. I know I didn't want to feed into false hope because we are taught that in nursing school. In hindsight, I now know that sometimes people have dreams that they take with them to the grave. They are entitled to those dreams right up to the very end. It is our job as health professionals to support their dreams with love and hope. Gary died two months later and several of the nurses and other staff members went to his funeral wake. As I walked in to give my condolences to his family, I could see Gary laid out in a gray suit and yes wearing his black bowtie to the ultimate interview with his God.

# 2009
# There Will Always Be Hope

When I let myself into Shakeema's room, all I can see are the green and yellow lights on her IV pump. I put my stethoscope around my neck, walk over to the bed and touch her hand to let her know I'm there. I go to the window, open the curtains and the early morning light spills across her bed. She slowly opens her brown eyes and looks over at me. I smile happily.

Shakeema's in the end-stage of AIDS and has had a lousy couple of days. She doesn't eat and sleeps most of the time. She has no family, just a few friends who visit in the evening, but only sometimes. Her time will come soon. When it will happen, is impossible to know. Some patients go quickly; others hold on for as long as they can. Everyone's different. As an AIDS Nurse, I make it a priority to help my patients in the end-stage of AIDS transition from life to death peacefully and with their dignity intact. Their lives have meaning regardless of how they contracted the virus.

A good nurse helps in the transition from life to death. In AIDS, there are no happy endings. However, it is important to know that each ending is as unique as the individual.

I walk over to Shakeema and gently take her hand.

"Good morning, Shakeema, how ya feeling, today?" I ask.

"Okay," she says softly.

I hear little squeaky sounds coming from her and I realize she is crying. "Shakeema, why the tears?"

She wipes her eyes and looks up at me, "You know, when I was younger, I did some modeling."

"I remember. You showed me your portfolio. I can still see you in that gold dress-with-the-slit up the side."

She manages a smile. "Dominick, can you get me the brush and the mirror," she says, barely audible. "I want to die pretty."

I go to her bedside table, take out the mirror, put it back and take out just the brush, instead. "Let me be your beautician," I offer.

"No, I have to do this myself, please."

I want to protect her from any more sadness and pain, but I know I must honor her request, so I hand her the mirror. She thanks me and holds it up to see her reflection.

"I don't look too bad, do I Dominick?"

"Shakeema, you're still beautiful."

She smiles back at me, puts the mirror down and closes her eyes. I can see she's tired, so I fluff up her pillow and turn the TV on low. The news stations are playing snippets of interviews with President Barack Obama and his first 100 days in office.

"Do you want to watch President Obama?" I ask her. She nods yes.

"That's good. Let's see what he has to say."

I sit in the sea foam green chair beside her bed and I see in her eyes that she wants to communicate but in her weakened state she just can't express her feelings. Together, we watch President Obama give a news conference. He stands at a podium with lots of American Flags behind him.

President Obama talks about the recession and how we have to tighten our belts. I wonder if he will mention anything about AIDS funding? Will he give us the changes he's promised? Will he give the AIDS community something to hope for?

As I sit here holding Shakeema's hand, I think back to the time when there was no HIV or AIDS, when beautiful young women like Shakeema were partying and having fun and didn't worry about death and dying.

My journey as an AIDS nurse began when HIV/AIDS was rampant, when I had already watched so many of my friends die from the disease. This is when the face of AIDS changed for me. Making the transition from caring for my gay friends with GRID/AIDS to caring for patients with AIDS at Broadway House. I have come to realize every person has a special journey in life: all very different, all very legitimate and all very real.

Along my journey as an AIDS Nurse, I gained experience in almost every aspect of AIDS Care. An AIDS activist before becoming a Registered Nurse, I worked in AIDS clinics, education and research, private practice and hospice/long term care. And in my free time, I facilitated three HIV/AIDS support groups. I am an AIDS-Certified Registered Nurse (ACRN) and a member of the

# My Journey as an AIDS Nurse

New Jersey Chapter of the Association of Nurses in AIDS Care, where I have held every position except secretary/treasurer.

Throughout my journey, I know I am better than "just a nurse". I am an AIDS Nurse, and I will follow this journey wherever it leads me.

One of the most important things I've learned on my journey is simple. To a Nurse, it should never matter why or how someone becomes sick. Everyone deserves to be treated with dignity so that when their time comes, they can leave this good earth feeling love, compassion and the loving touch of someone holding their hand.

*This book is dedicated ...*

*...to Bob.* I know God is with me in all I do. He gave me a life partner in Bob Buhr who has given me unconditional love for many years. No one deserves this dedication more than he does.

*...to my family.* God gave me wonderful caring parents who gave me many gifts in life; especially the gift of charity to others. He gave me a family who, regardless of our vast differences in opinion, still hold love in our hearts for each other, as we walk our own journey. For all of my family, extended families, friends, and my patients who died from AIDS and other illnesses.

Thank you for being in my life.

*...to my friends,* Roro, Ms. Jewel, Reymundo, Ron, and Anthony who all inspire me.

My heart is happy and my soul is light because so many people I know and many I have met along my journey have supported my endeavors especially Arlene & Marty G and family, Tina, Florence Holmes, Robert Mason, Lou Squitieri, Virginia Neilly, Ruth M, Alice G, Mom Bax, and the volunteers, members and supporters of Positive Connection

*...to Christ Hospital School of Nursing educators and staff,* especially George Hebert, Carol Fasano, Emily Marcelo, Rose O'Connor, Dawn Gerbino, Barbara Davey

**...to my Clergy support**, especially Episcopal Bishop of Newark, NJ John Shelby Spong, Father Steven Giovangelo and Father Peter DeFranco

*...to all the Nurses* who were on duty when no one knew what AIDS or GRID were, and to all Nurses throughout the world, you are the heroes of my journey and the journey of every patient in your care.

*...to all of my friends, & patients who died from AIDS or live with it still and those who support them.*

*and to* **my friend** Sally Deering. Many people heard my stories and said I should write a book.

Sally saw to it that I followed through.

*I love you all...*

# About the Authors

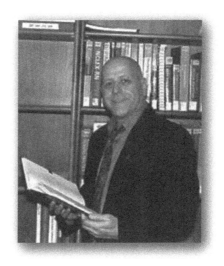

*Authors' Note: Some of the names in this book were changed to protect privacy and uphold confidentiality*

**D**ominick P. Varsalone was raised in New Jersey, the fourth of five children born to Roman Catholic parents. He attended Catholic schools through the eighth grade, and after high school, he joined his father working in the railroad industry, where he experienced persecution for being gay.

*My Journey as an AIDS Nurse* is Varsalone's first book. He has previously published three books of poetry and also presented at the International AIDS Conference in Bangkok, Thailand, in 2004.

As a nurse, he was honored with the Bishop of Newark Award for compassion, which led to his introduction to Bishop John Shelby Spong, who has since had a strong and positive influence on Varsalone's religious views. He has won numerous other awards as an AIDS nurse and has been asked to speak to various groups on the subject of HIV/AIDS empowerment.

Varsalone lives in Asheville, North Carolina, with his husband, Robert Buhr.

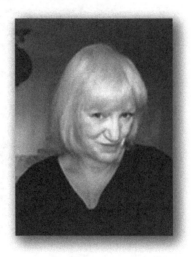

**Sally Deering** is an award-winning journalist and playwright, a filmmaker, and author of *The Apple that Fell from the Orange Tree*, (Kindle Direct Publishing) available on Amazon.com. Sally lives in Weehawken, New Jersey, where she gets much of her inspiration looking out at the Manhattan Skyline. To contact Sally, email: SallyDeer@gmail.com

**Cover illustration: Mendoza Productions, Weehawken, NJ
fermin_mendoza13@yahoo.com**

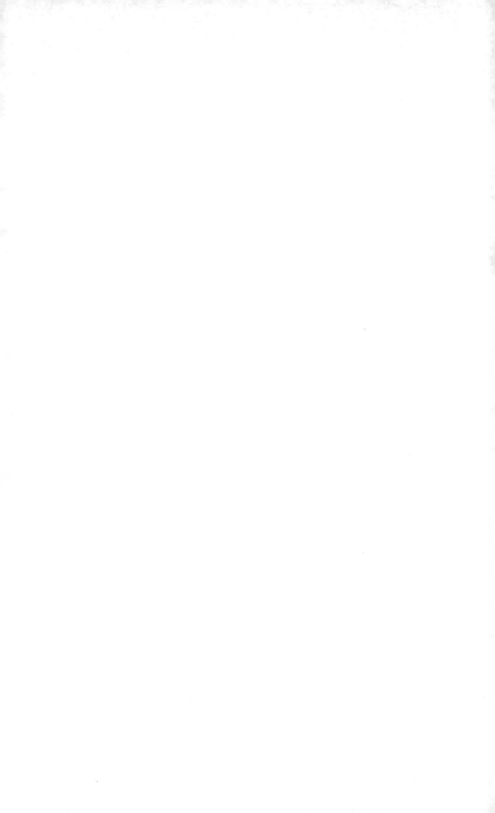